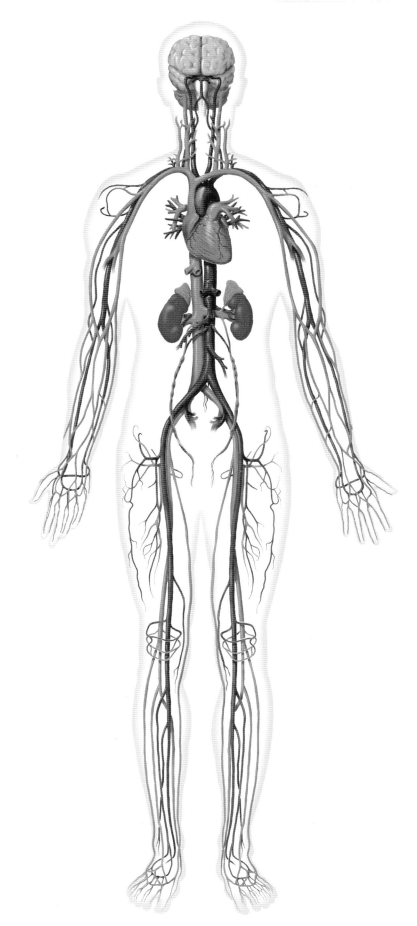

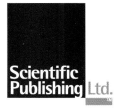

ISBN13: 978-1-932922-95-0   Item# ANAT-25

Published in the United States by: Scientific Publishing Ltd. 129 Joey Drive, Elk Grove Village, IL 60007

Printed in Korea

Individual chart titles are available at www.scientificpublishing.com

The Skeletal System

Axial skeleton
Appendicular skeleton

Key of abbreviations
b. Bone   Vertebrae:
l. Ligament   **C** Cervical
ll. Ligaments   **T** Thoracic
t. Tendon   **L** Lumbar

Anterior view

Frontal b.
Supraorbital notch
Lesser wing of sphenoid b.
Greater wing of sphenoid b.
Temporal b.
Inferior orbital fissure
Infraorbital foramen
Inferior nasal concha
Maxilla
Mental foramen
Parietal b.
Nasal b.
Ethmoid b.
Superior orbital fissure
Orbit
Zygomatic b.
Lacrimal b.
Nasal septum
Vomer
Mandible

Anterior longitudinal l.
Jugular notch
Manubrium of sternum
Scapular notch
Coracoid process
Acromion
Greater tubercle
Lesser tubercle
Intertubercular groove
Head of humerus
Subscapular fossa
Scapula
Nutrient foramen
Humerus
Deltoid tuberosity
True ribs (1–7)
False ribs (8–12)

Hyoid b.
Sternoclavicular l.
Costoclavicular l.
Clavicle
Acromioclavicular l.
Coracoacromial l.
Supraspinatus t.
Coracohumeral l.
Transverse humeral l.
Articular capsule
Subscapularis t.
Tendon of long head of biceps
Body of sternum
Radiate ll.
Xiphoid process
Costal cartilages
Interchondral ll.

Medial epicondyle
Coronoid fossa
Lateral epicondyle
Capitulum
Trochlea
Head of radius
Ulnar tuberosity
Radial tuberosity
Coronoid process
Floating ribs
Sacral promontory
Radius
Ulna

Anterior longitudinal l.
Ulnar collateral l.
Radial collateral l.
Annular l.
Articular capsule
Iliolumbar l.

Ilium
Iliac crest
Anterior superior iliac spine
Spine of ischium
Anterior inferior iliac spine
Head of femur
Greater trochanter
Obturator foramen
Carpal bones:
Lunate
Scaphoid
Capitate
Trapezium
Trapezoid
Proximal phalanx
Metacarpals
Distal phalanx

Anterior sacroiliac l.
Anterior sacrococcygeal l.
Sacrotuberous l.
Sacrospinous l.
Inguinal l.
Iliofemoral l.
Pubofemoral l.
Obturator membrane
Interosseous membrane
Palmar ulnocarpal l.
Palmar radiocarpal l.
Radial collateral l.
Palmar carpometacarpal ll.
Palmar metacarpal ll.
Carpal bones:
Pisiform
Hamate
Triquetral
Lesser trochanter
Coccyx
Pubis
Pubic symphysis
Arcuate pubic l.
Superior pubic l.
Proximal phalanges
Middle phalanges
Distal phalanges
Ulnar collateral l.
Pisometacarpal l.
Pisohamate l.
Capitotriquetral l.
Deep transverse metacarpal l.
Articular capsules with palmar ll.
Articular capsules
Femur

Vertebral column
(Lateral view)

Atlas (C1)
Axis (C2)
Cervical vertebrae (C1–C7)
Cervical curve
C7
T1
Intervertebral discs
Thoracic vertebrae (T1–T12)
Thoracic curve
Foveae for ribs
T12
L1
Lumbar vertebrae (L1–L5)
Lumbar curve
Intervertebral foramina
L5
Sacrum
Pelvic curve
Coccyx

Posterior view

Parietal b.
Occipital b.
Temporal b.
Posterior atlanto-occipital membrane
Ligamenta flava
Mandible
Articular capsules
Superior costotransverse ll.
Acromioclavicular l.
Superior transverse scapular l.
Infraspinatus t.
Teres minor t.
Articular capsule
Inferior transverse scapular l.

Mastoid process
Atlas (C1)
Axis (C2)
Transverse processes
Lateral masses
C7 spinous process
Lateral costotransverse ll.
Clavicle
Supraspinous fossa
Scapular notch
Spine of scapula
Acromion
Head of humerus
Greater tubercle
Infraspinous fossa
Scapula
Humerus
Deltoid tuberosity

Articular capsule
Radial collateral l.
Annular l.
Supraspinous ll.
Iliolumbar l.
Posterior sacroiliac l.
Long posterior sacroiliac l.
Posterior sacrococcygeal l.
Sacrospinous l.
Iliofemoral l.
Ischiofemoral l.
Interosseous membrane
Ulnar collateral l.
Dorsal radiocarpal l.
Medial epicondyle
Olecranon fossa
Lateral epicondyle
Olecranon
Groove for ulnar nerve
Head of radius
Head of ulna
L1
Sacral tuberosity
Iliac crest
Ilium
Posterior superior iliac spine
Sacrum
Greater sciatic notch
Ischium
Head of femur
Greater trochanter
Intertrochanteric crest
Radius
Ulna
Dorsal ulnocarpal l.
Ulnar collateral l.
Dorsal carpometacarpal ll.
Dorsal metacarpal ll.
Sacrotuberous l.
Obturator membrane
Coccyx
Ischial tuberosity
Obturator foramen
Pubis
Carpal bones:
Lunate
Triquetral
Hamate
Metacarpals
Proximal phalanges
Middle phalanges
Distal phalanges
Carpal bones:
Scaphoid
Capitate
Trapezoid
Trapezium
Proximal phalanx
Distal phalanx
Femur
Linea aspera

Bones of the right ear
(Medial view)

Malleus
Anterior process
Lenticular process
Handle
Anterior limb
Incus
Short process
Long process
Stapes

Compact bone

Lamellae
Canaliculi
Lacuna
Osteon
Osteocyte
Arteriole, venule and nerve in central canal
Lamellae
Spongy bone
Interstitial systems
Osteons
Central canals
Periosteum

Common names of bones

Common name	Refers to the:
Collar bone	Clavicle
Breast bone	Sternum
Rib cage	Sternum, ribs, costal cartilages, and thoracic vertebrae
Shoulder blade	Scapula
Elbow bone	Olecranon of ulna
Funny bone	Ulnar nerve as it wraps around the humerus at the elbow
Backbone	Vertebral column
Spine	Vertebral column
Tail bone	Coccyx
Hip bone	Ilium
Thigh bone	Femur
Kneecap	Patella
Shin bone	Tibia

Quadriceps femoris t.
Lateral epicondyle
Lateral condyles
Head of fibula
Medial patellar retinaculum
Medial epicondyle
Patella
Medial condyles
Patellar l.
Tibial collateral l.
Fibular collateral l.
Lateral patellar retinaculum
Tibial tuberosity
Tibia
Fibula
Interosseous membrane
Lateral malleolus
Medial malleolus
Tarsal bones:
Navicular
Intermediate cuneiform
Medial cuneiform
Calcaneus
Tarsal bones:
Talus
Lateral cuneiform
Cuboid
Deltoid l.
Anterior tibiofibular l.
Dorsal cuneonavicular l.
Dorsal tarso-metatarsal l.
Dorsal metatarsal l.
Articular capsules

Female pelvis
Anterior view

Anterior superior iliac spines farther apart
Pelvic inlet round or oval
Pubic symphysis shallower, shorter
Obturator foramen triangular
Pubic arch obtuse (greater than 90°)
Processes less prominent
Superior View
Pelvic outlet wider

Male pelvis
Anterior view

Anterior superior iliac spines closer together
Pelvic inlet heart-shaped
Pubic symphysis deeper, longer
Obturator foramen oval
Pubic arch acute (less than 90°)
Processes more prominent
Superior View
Pelvic outlet narrower

Bones and ligaments of the right foot
(Plantar view)

1 Distal phalanges
2 Middle phalanges
3 Proximal phalanges
4 Metatarsal bones I to V
5 Sesamoid bones*
6 Lateral cuneiform b.
7 Intermediate cuneiform b.
8 Medial cuneiform b.
9 Cuboid b.
10 Navicular b.
11 Talus
12 Calcaneus
13 Articular capsules
14 Deep transverse metatarsal l.
15 Plantar metatarsal ll.
16 Peroneus longus t.
17 Plantar calcaneocuboid (short plantar) l.
18 Long plantar l.
19 Plantar tarsometatarsal ll.
20 Plantar calcaneonavicular (spring) l.
21 Tibialis posterior t.

*A **sesamoid bone** is a bone that forms in a tendon over a joint. The patellae (kneecaps) are large sesamoid bones that all people have. Most people have extra, much smaller sesamoid bones near other joints, often in the hands and feet.

Cross-section of the femur

Anterior cruciate l.
Posterior menisco-femoral l.
Fibular collateral l.
Lateral meniscus
Posterior cruciate l.
Articular capsule, cut
Medial epicondyle
Tibial collateral l.
Medial meniscus
Medial condyles
Intercondylar eminence
Intercondylar fossa
Lateral epicondyle
Lateral condyles
Head of fibula
Interosseous membrane
Tibia
Fibula
Medial malleolus
Lateral malleolus
Talus
Calcaneus
Posterior tibiofibular l.
Posterior talofibular l.
Calcaneofibular l.
Deltoid l.
Calcaneal (Achilles) l.

Periosteum
Compact bone
Diaphysis
Nutrient artery in nutrient foramen
Medullary cavity
Periosteum
Compact bone
Endosteum
Yellow bone marrow
Spongy bone
Epiphyseal line
Epiphysis
Articular cartilage
Red bone marrow
Red blood cell
Platelets
White blood cell

PLATE 1

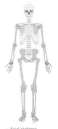

The Vertebral Column

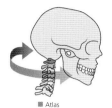

■ Axial skeleton
■ Appendicular skeleton

The spine

The spine is a column of 26 bones that extends from the base of the skull to the pelvis and supports the head, shoulders and chest. The spine also protects the **spinal cord**, a long, fragile structure composed of nerves that transmit signals between the brain and body, enabling movement and sensation. As the spinal cord passes through the **vertebral foramen** at the center of the vertebrae, pairs of **spinal nerves** (roots) enter and emerge between the vertebral spaces, connecting with nerves throughout the body. The spine is held in place by **ligaments and tendons** that attach to bony processes at the back (posterior) of the vertebrae and connect to the muscles of the back.

Atlas and axis

The uppermost vertebrae of the spine play an important role in the motion and flexibility of the head. The atlas keeps the head supported and enables up and down (nodding) motion while preventing twisting. Articulation with the axis allows side-to-side (rotating) movement of the head. Powerful muscles connected to the spinous process of the axis control the position of both the head and neck.

■ Atlas
■ Axis

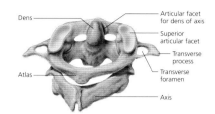

Dens
Atlas
Articular facet for dens of axis
Superior articular facet
Transverse process
Transverse foramen
Axis

The types of vertebrae

Cervical vertebrae
Seven cervical vertebrae (C1–C7), beginning with the atlas and axis, form the upper portion of the spine. Nerves controlling the neck, upper body and arms pass through the foramen of the cervical vertebrae, while arteries carrying blood to the brain pass through special openings in the bony side processes.

Thoracic vertebrae
The middle of the spine is made up of twelve thoracic vertebrae (T1–T12) that attach to the ribs and help support the area between the neck and diaphragm. The thoracic spine has more limited motion than the upper or lower regions of the spine.

Lumbar vertebrae
The lumbar vertebrae are the largest bones in the spine and carry the majority of the body's weight. There are five lumbar vertebrae (L1–L5), although six may also be present. Five pairs of nerves pass through the lumbar spine to control the movement and sensory functions of the lower body.

Cervical vertebrae

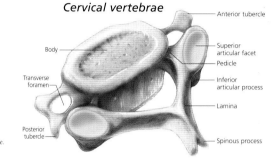

Anterior tubercle
Body
Superior articular facet
Pedicle
Transverse foramen
Inferior articular process
Lamina
Posterior tubercle
Spinous process

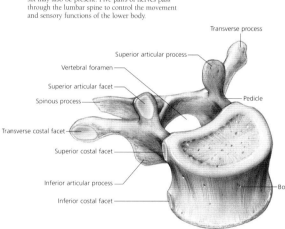

Transverse process
Superior articular process
Vertebral foramen
Superior articular facet
Spinous process
Transverse costal facet
Superior costal facet
Inferior articular process
Inferior costal facet
Pedicle
Body

Spinal cord
Spinal nerves

Thoracic vertebrae

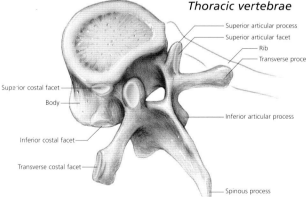

Superior articular process
Superior articular facet
Rib
Transverse process
Superior costal facet
Body
Inferior articular process
Inferior costal facet
Transverse costal facet
Spinous process

Lumbar vertebrae

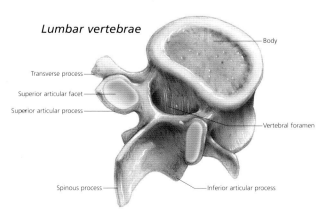

Body
Transverse process
Superior articular facet
Superior articular process
Vertebral foramen
Spinous process
Inferior articular process

The sacrum and coccyx

The spine ends with the distinctly shaped sacrum and coccyx bones. The triangular sacrum contains five fused vertebrae and adds strength and stability to the pelvis. The tail-shaped coccyx includes four fused vertebrae and connects several large muscles to the lower spine.

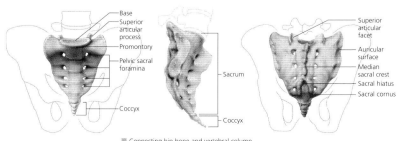

Base
Superior articular process
Promontory
Pelvic sacral foramina
Coccyx
Sacrum
Coccyx
Superior articular facet
Auricular surface
Median sacral crest
Sacral hiatus
Sacral cornua

■ Connecting hip bone and vertebral column

C1
C7
T1
T12
L1
L5

Cervical vertebrae
Cervical vertebrae (C1–C7)
Thoracic vertebrae
Thoracic vertebrae (T1–T12)
Lumbar vertebrae
Lumbar vertebrae (L1–L5)
Pelvic curve

Vertebral column
(Anterior view)

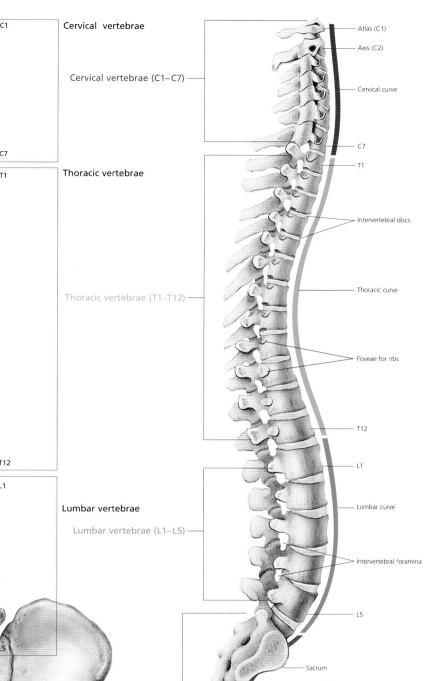

Atlas (C1)
Axis (C2)
Cervical curve
C7
T1
Intervertebral discs
Thoracic curve
Foveae for ribs
T12
L1
Lumbar curve
Intervertebral foramina
L5
Sacrum
Pelvic curve
Coccyx

Vertebral column
(Lateral view)

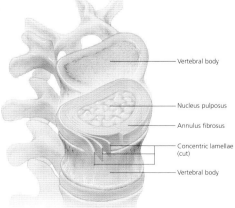

Vertebral body
Nucleus pulposus
Annulus fibrosus
Concentric lamellae (cut)
Vertebral body

Intervertebral disc

Intervertebral discs

The spinal column is protected from within by intervertebral discs. Each round, flat disc is composed of a tough outer ligament that holds the disc together and a resilient, fluid-filled center that acts as a shock absorber.

The intervertebral discs play a critical role in protecting the spine from injury, preventing the vertebrae from rubbing together and providing the spine with flexibility.

PLATE 2

The Skull

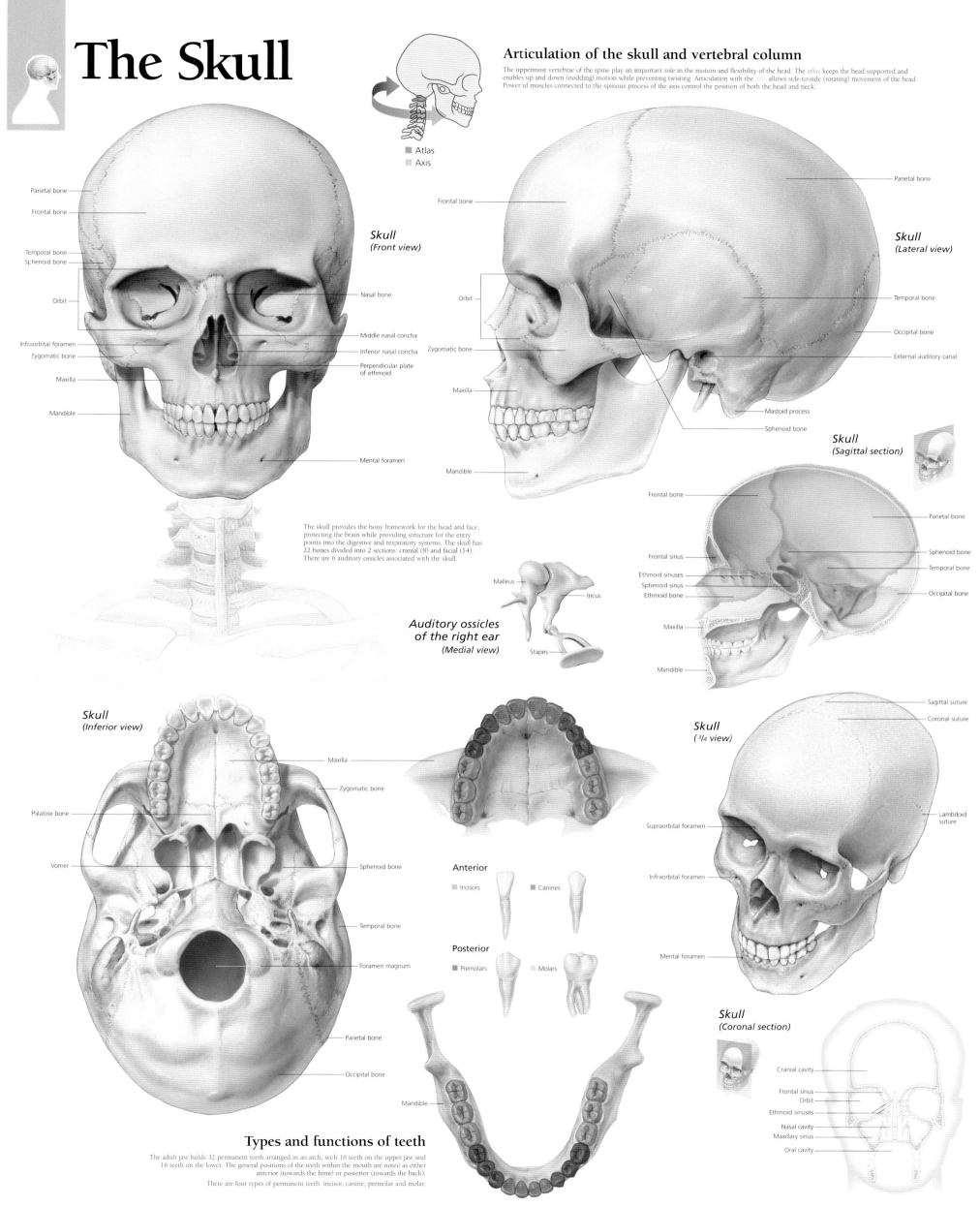

Articulation of the skull and vertebral column

The uppermost vertebrae of the spine play an important role in the motion and flexibility of the head. The atlas keeps the head supported and enables up and down (nodding) motion while preventing twisting. Articulation with the axis allows side-to-side (rotating) movement of the head. Powerful muscles connected to the spinous process of the axis control the position of both the head and neck.

- Atlas
- Axis

Skull
(Front view)

Parietal bone
Frontal bone
Temporal bone
Sphenoid bone
Orbit
Infraorbital foramen
Zygomatic bone
Maxilla
Mandible

Nasal bone
Middle nasal concha
Inferior nasal concha
Perpendicular plate of ethmoid
Mental foramen

Skull
(Lateral view)

Frontal bone
Orbit
Zygomatic bone
Maxilla
Mandible

Parietal bone
Temporal bone
Occipital bone
External auditory canal
Mastoid process
Sphenoid bone

The skull provides the bony framework for the head and face, protecting the brain while providing structure for the entry points into the digestive and respiratory systems. The skull has 22 bones divided into 2 sections: cranial (8) and facial (14). There are 6 auditory ossicles associated with the skull.

Auditory ossicles of the right ear
(Medial view)

Malleus
Incus
Stapes

Skull
(Sagittal section)

Frontal bone
Frontal sinus
Ethmoid sinuses
Sphenoid sinus
Ethmoid bone
Maxilla
Mandible

Parietal bone
Sphenoid bone
Temporal bone
Occipital bone

Skull
(Inferior view)

Palatine bone
Vomer
Maxilla
Zygomatic bone
Sphenoid bone
Temporal bone
Foramen magnum
Parietal bone
Occipital bone

Skull
(³/₄ view)

Sagittal suture
Coronal suture
Supraorbital foramen
Infraorbital foramen
Mental foramen
Lambdoid suture

Types and functions of teeth

The adult jaw holds 32 permanent teeth arranged in an arch, with 16 teeth on the upper jaw and 16 teeth on the lower. The general positions of the teeth within the mouth are noted as either anterior (towards the front) or posterior (towards the back).

There are four types of permanent teeth: incisor, canine, premolar and molar.

Anterior
- Incisors
- Canines

Posterior
- Premolars
- Molars

Mandible

Skull
(Coronal section)

Cranial cavity
Frontal sinus
Orbit
Ethmoid sinuses
Nasal cavity
Maxillary sinus
Oral cavity

PLATE 3

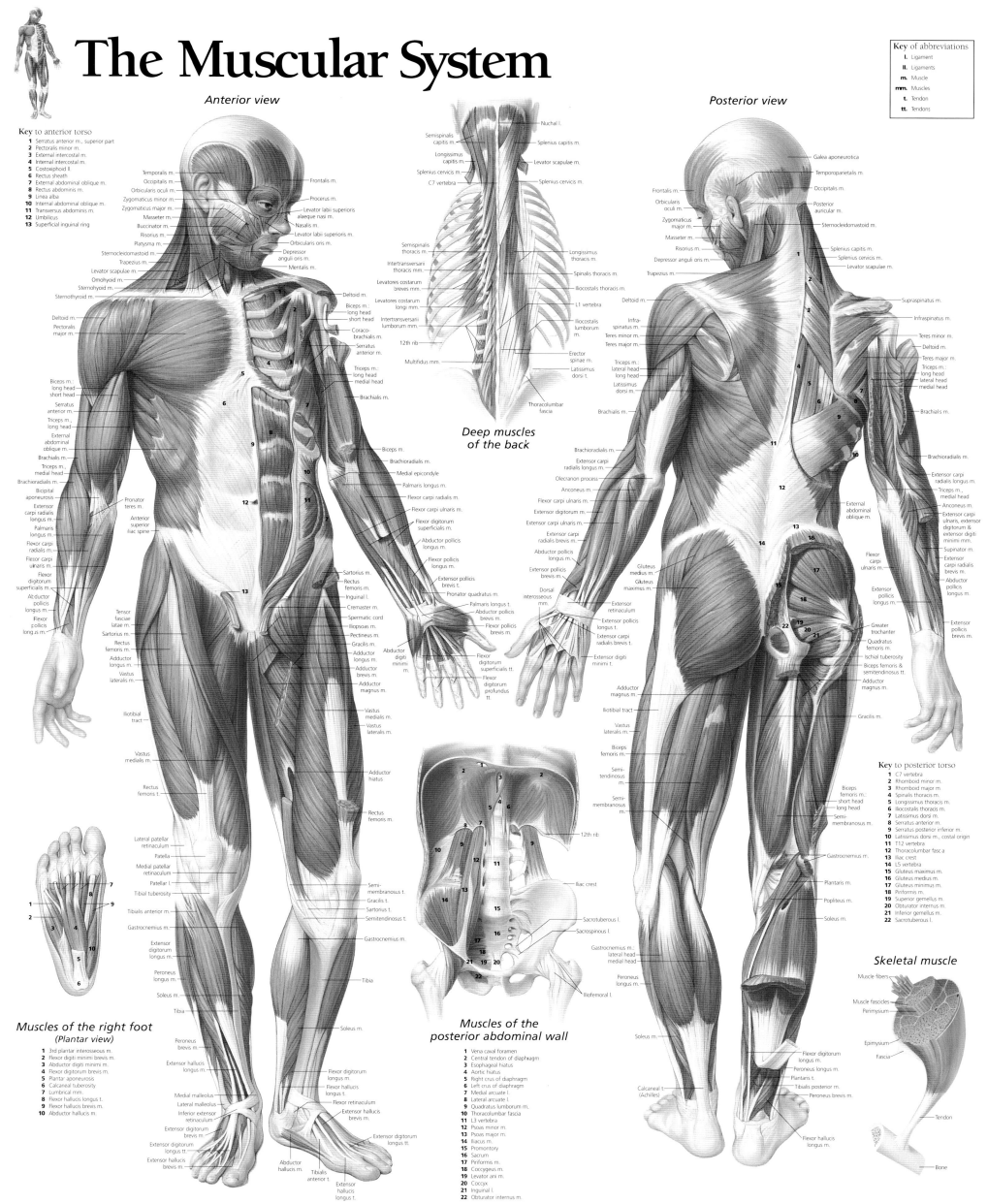

The Muscular System

Anterior view

Posterior view

©Scientific Publishing Ltd., Elk Grove Village, IL, USA
#1100

PLATE 4

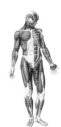

The Hip & Knee

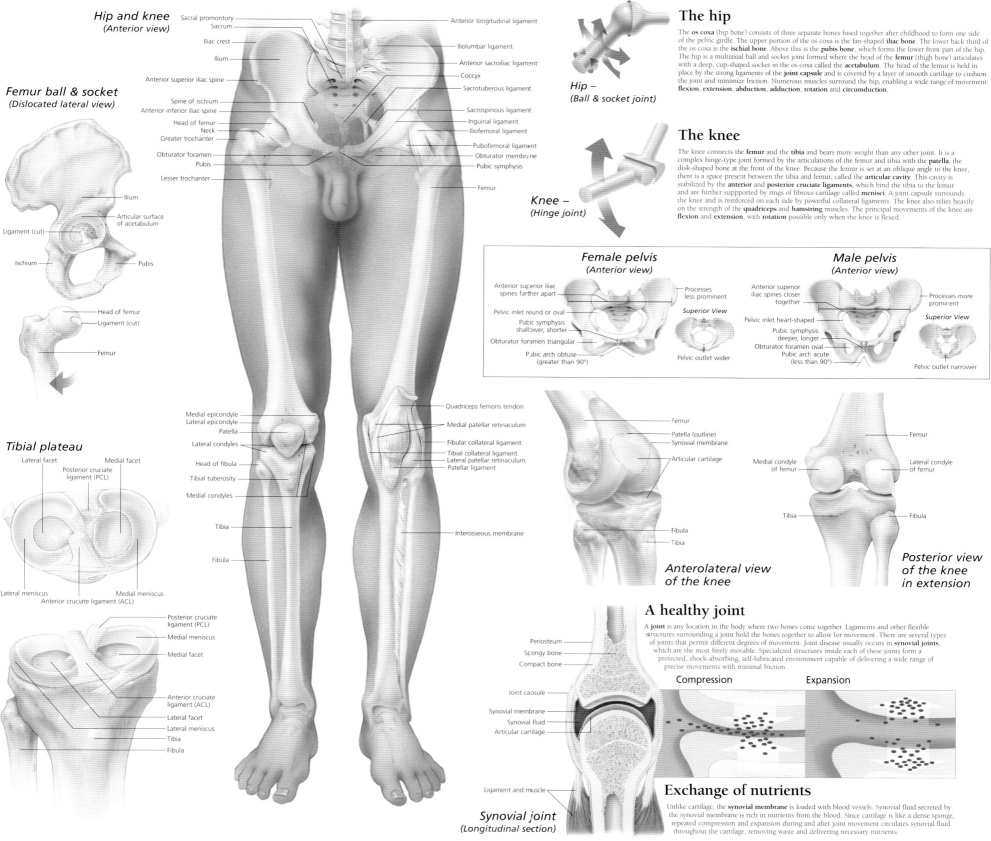

Hip and knee
(Anterior view)

- Sacral promontory
- Sacrum
- Iliac crest
- Ilium
- Anterior superior iliac spine
- Spine of ischium
- Anterior inferior iliac spine
- Head of femur
- Neck
- Greater trochanter
- Obturator foramen
- Pubis
- Lesser trochanter

- Anterior longitudinal ligament
- Iliolumbar ligament
- Anterior sacroiliac ligament
- Coccyx
- Sacrotuberous ligament
- Sacrospinous ligament
- Inguinal ligament
- Iliofemoral ligament
- Pubofemoral ligament
- Obturator membrane
- Pubic symphysis
- Femur

Femur ball & socket
(Dislocated lateral view)

- Ilium
- Articular surface of acetabulum
- Ligament (cut)
- Ischium
- Pubis
- Head of femur
- Ligament (cut)
- Femur

Tibial plateau

- Lateral facet
- Medial facet
- Posterior cruciate ligament (PCL)
- Lateral meniscus
- Medial meniscus
- Anterior cruciate ligament (ACL)

- Posterior cruciate ligament (PCL)
- Medial meniscus
- Medial facet
- Anterior cruciate ligament (ACL)
- Lateral facet
- Lateral meniscus
- Tibia
- Fibula

- Medial epicondyle
- Lateral epicondyle
- Patella
- Lateral condyles
- Head of fibula
- Tibial tuberosity
- Medial condyles
- Tibia
- Fibula

- Quadriceps femoris tendon
- Medial patellar retinaculum
- Fibular collateral ligament
- Tibial collateral ligament
- Lateral patellar retinaculum
- Patellar ligament
- Interosseous membrane

The hip

The **os coxa** (hip bone) consists of three separate bones fused together after childhood to form one side of the pelvic girdle. The upper portion of the os coxa is the fan-shaped **iliac bone**. The lower back third of the os coxa is the **ischial bone**. Above this is the **pubis bone**, which forms the lower front part of the hip. The hip is a multiaxial ball and socket joint formed where the head of the **femur** (thigh bone) articulates with a deep, cup-shaped socket in the os coxa called the **acetabulum**. The head of the femur is held in place by the strong ligaments of the **joint capsule** and is covered by a layer of smooth cartilage to cushion the joint and minimize friction. Numerous muscles surround the hip, enabling a wide range of movement: **flexion**, **extension**, **abduction**, **adduction**, **rotation** and **circumduction**.

Hip –
(Ball & socket joint)

The knee

The knee connects the **femur** and the **tibia** and bears more weight than any other joint. It is a complex hinge-type joint formed by the articulations of the femur and tibia with the **patella**, the disk-shaped bone at the front of the knee. Because the femur is set at an oblique angle to the knee, there is a space present between the tibia and femur, called the **articular cavity**. This cavity is stabilized by the **anterior** and **posterior cruciate ligaments**, which bind the tibia to the femur and are further suppported by rings of fibrous cartilage called **menisci**. A joint capsule surrounds the knee and is reinforced on each side by powerful collateral ligaments. The knee also relies heavily on the strength of the **quadriceps** and **hamstring** muscles. The principal movements of the knee are **flexion** and **extension**, with **rotation** possible only when the knee is flexed.

Knee –
(Hinge joint)

Female pelvis
(Anterior view)

- Anterior superior iliac spines farther apart
- Processes less prominent
- Pelvic inlet round or oval
- Pubic symphysis shallower, shorter
- Obturator foramen triangular
- Pubic arch obtuse (greater than 90°)
- *Superior View*
- Pelvic outlet wider

Male pelvis
(Anterior view)

- Anterior superior iliac spines closer together
- Processes more prominent
- Pelvic inlet heart-shaped
- Pubic symphysis deeper, longer
- Obturator foramen oval
- Pubic arch acute (less than 90°)
- *Superior View*
- Pelvic outlet narrower

Anterolateral view of the knee

- Femur
- Patella (outline)
- Synovial membrane
- Articular cartilage
- Fibula
- Tibia

Posterior view of the knee in extension

- Femur
- Medial condyle of femur
- Lateral condyle of femur
- Tibia
- Fibula

A healthy joint

A **joint** is any location in the body where two bones come together. Ligaments and other flexible structures surrounding a joint hold the bones together to allow for movement. There are several types of joints that permit different degrees of movement. Joint disease usually occurs in **synovial joints**, which are the most freely movable. Specialized structures inside each of these joints form a protected, shock-absorbing, self-lubricated environment capable of delivering a wide range of precise movements with minimal friction.

- Periosteum
- Spongy bone
- Compact bone
- Joint capsule
- Synovial membrane
- Synovial fluid
- Articular cartilage
- Ligament and muscle

Synovial joint
(Longitudinal section)

Compression

Expansion

Exchange of nutrients

Unlike cartilage, the **synovial membrane** is loaded with blood vessels. Synovial fluid secreted by the synovial membrane is rich in nutrients from the blood. Since cartilage is like a dense sponge, repeated compression and expansion during and after joint movement circulates synovial fluid throughout the cartilage, removing waste and delivering necessary nutrients.

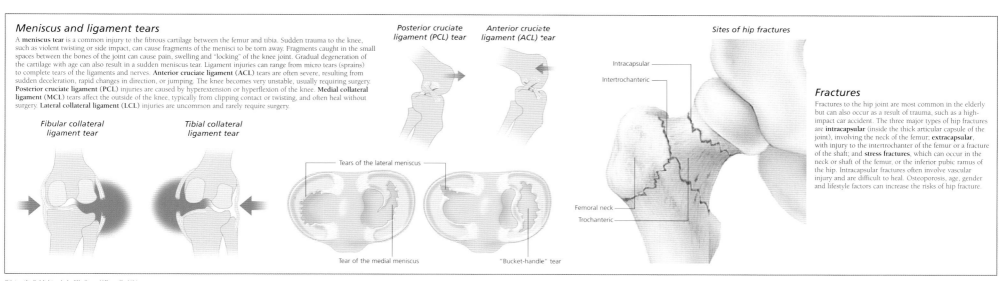

Meniscus and ligament tears

A **meniscus tear** is a common injury to the fibrous cartilage between the femur and tibia. Sudden trauma to the knee, such as violent twisting or side impact, can cause fragments of the menisci to be torn away. Fragments caught in the small spaces between the bones of the joint can cause pain, swelling and "locking" of the knee joint. Gradual degeneration of the cartilage with age can also result in a sudden meniscus tear. Ligament injuries can range from micro tears (sprains) to complete tears of the ligaments and nerves. **Anterior cruciate ligament (ACL)** tears are often severe, resulting from sudden deceleration, rapid changes in direction, or jumping. The knee becomes very unstable, usually requiring surgery. **Posterior cruciate ligament (PCL)** injuries are caused by hyperextension or hyperflexion of the knee. **Medial collateral ligament (MCL)** tears affect the outside of the knee, typically from clipping contact or twisting, and often heal without surgery. **Lateral collateral ligament (LCL)** injuries are uncommon and rarely require surgery.

Posterior cruciate ligament (PCL) tear

Anterior cruciate ligament (ACL) tear

Fibular collateral ligament tear

Tibial collateral ligament tear

- Tears of the lateral meniscus
- Tear of the medial meniscus
- "Bucket-handle" tear

Sites of hip fractures

- Intracapsular
- Intertrochanteric
- Femoral neck
- Trochanteric

Fractures

Fractures to the hip joint are most common in the elderly but can also occur as a result of trauma, such as a high-impact car accident. The three major types of hip fractures are **intracapsular** (inside the thick articular capsule of the joint), involving the neck of the femur; **extracapsular**, with injury to the intertrochanter of the femur or a fracture of the shaft; and **stress fractures**, which can occur in the neck or shaft of the femur, or the inferior pubic ramus of the hip. Intracapsular fractures often involve vascular injury and are difficult to heal. Osteoporosis, age, gender and lifestyle factors can increase the risks of hip fracture.

PLATE 5

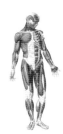

The Shoulder & Elbow

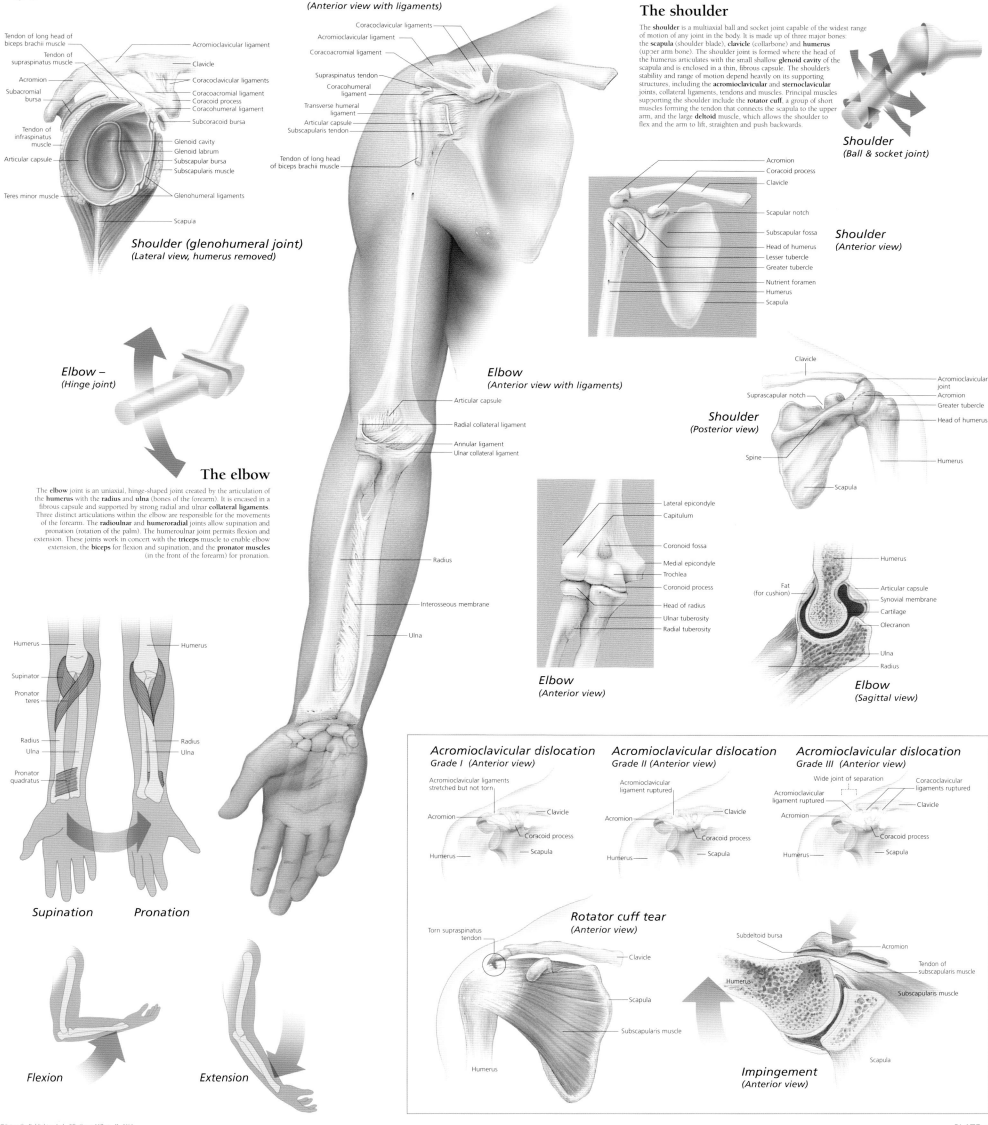

Shoulder
(Anterior view with ligaments)

Tendon of long head of biceps brachii muscle
Tendon of supraspinatus muscle
Acromion
Subacromial bursa
Tendon of infraspinatus muscle
Articular capsule
Teres minor muscle
Acromioclavicular ligament
Clavicle
Coracoclavicular ligaments
Coracoacromial ligament
Coracoid process
Coracohumeral ligament
Subcoracoid bursa
Glenoid cavity
Glenoid labrum
Subscapular bursa
Subscapularis muscle
Glenohumeral ligaments
Scapula

Shoulder (glenohumeral joint)
(Lateral view, humerus removed)

Coracoclavicular ligaments
Acromioclavicular ligament
Coracoacromial ligament
Supraspinatus tendon
Coracohumeral ligament
Transverse humeral ligament
Articular capsule
Subscapularis tendon
Tendon of long head of biceps brachii muscle

The shoulder

The **shoulder** is a multiaxial ball and socket joint capable of the widest range of motion of any joint in the body. It is made up of three major bones: the **scapula** (shoulder blade), **clavicle** (collarbone) and **humerus** (upper arm bone). The shoulder joint is formed where the head of the humerus articulates with the small shallow **glenoid cavity** of the scapula and is enclosed in a thin, fibrous capsule. The shoulder's stability and range of motion depend heavily on its supporting structures, including the **acromioclavicular** and **sternoclavicular** joints, collateral ligaments, tendons and muscles. Principal muscles supporting the shoulder include the **rotator cuff**, a group of short muscles forming the tendon that connects the scapula to the upper arm, and the large **deltoid** muscle, which allows the shoulder to flex and the arm to lift, straighten and push backwards.

Shoulder
(Ball & socket joint)

Acromion
Coracoid process
Clavicle
Scapular notch
Subscapular fossa
Head of humerus
Lesser tubercle
Greater tubercle
Nutrient foramen
Humerus
Scapula

Shoulder
(Anterior view)

Elbow –
(Hinge joint)

Elbow
(Anterior view with ligaments)

Articular capsule
Radial collateral ligament
Annular ligament
Ulnar collateral ligament

Clavicle
Suprascapular notch
Spine
Acromioclavicular joint
Acromion
Greater tubercle
Head of humerus
Humerus
Scapula

Shoulder
(Posterior view)

The elbow

The **elbow** joint is an uniaxial, hinge-shaped joint created by the articulation of the **humerus** with the **radius** and **ulna** (bones of the forearm). It is encased in a fibrous capsule and supported by strong radial and ulnar **collateral ligaments**. Three distinct articulations within the elbow are responsible for the movements of the forearm. The **radioulnar** and **humeroradial** joints allow supination and pronation (rotation of the palm). The humeroulnar joint permits flexion and extension. These joints work in concert with the **triceps** muscle to enable elbow extension, the **biceps** for flexion and supination, and the **pronator muscles** (in the front of the forearm) for pronation.

Radius
Interosseous membrane
Ulna

Lateral epicondyle
Capitulum
Coronoid fossa
Medial epicondyle
Trochlea
Coronoid process
Head of radius
Ulnar tuberosity
Radial tuberosity

Elbow
(Anterior view)

Humerus
Fat (for cushion)
Articular capsule
Synovial membrane
Cartilage
Olecranon
Ulna
Radius

Elbow
(Sagittal view)

Humerus
Supinator
Pronator teres
Radius
Ulna
Pronator quadratus
Humerus
Radius
Ulna

Supination   **Pronation**

Flexion   **Extension**

Acromioclavicular dislocation
Grade I *(Anterior view)*

Acromioclavicular ligaments stretched but not torn
Acromion
Clavicle
Coracoid process
Humerus
Scapula

Acromioclavicular dislocation
Grade II *(Anterior view)*

Acromioclavicular ligament ruptured
Acromion
Clavicle
Coracoid process
Humerus
Scapula

Acromioclavicular dislocation
Grade III *(Anterior view)*

Wide joint of separation
Acromioclavicular ligament ruptured
Acromion
Coracoclavicular ligaments ruptured
Clavicle
Coracoid process
Humerus
Scapula

Rotator cuff tear
(Anterior view)

Torn supraspinatus tendon
Clavicle
Scapula
Subscapularis muscle
Humerus

Impingement
(Anterior view)

Subdeltoid bursa
Acromion
Tendon of subscapularis muscle
Subscapularis muscle
Humerus
Scapula

The Foot & Ankle

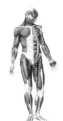

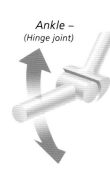

Ankle –
(Hinge joint)

The foot and ankle

The foot and ankle form a complex structure that includes 33 joints, 26 bones and more than 100 muscles, tendons and ligaments. The feet and ankles work together to provide the body with support, balance and mobility.

Structurally, the **foot** is divided into three sections. The **forefoot** plays a major role in weight-bearing and balance and contains the long bones of the foot (**metatarsals**) and the toes (**phalanges**), which are connected at the ball of the foot by five metatarsal phalangeal joints. The **midfoot** contains five interlocking **tarsal bones** (cuboid, navicular, and 3 cuneiform) that form the arch of the foot. It is connected to the forefoot and hindfoot by muscles and the **plantar fascia** ligament, an important structure that stabilizes the foot and helps maintain the arch. Two additional tarsal bones make up the **hindfoot**. The **calcaneus** (heel) is the largest, strongest bone in the foot and the site of attachment for the powerful **Achilles tendon**. The **talus** (astragalus) sits above the calcaneus and between the lower ends of the leg bones (**tibia** and **fibula**) to form the ankle joint. The talus is involved in multiple planes of movement and is responsible for transferring weight and pressure from the leg to the foot.

The ankle joint itself is a uniaxial, hinge-type joint capable of both upwards (**dorsiflexion**) and downwards (**plantarflexion**) motion. Limited rotation, abduction and adduction is also possible. The ankle joint is protected by a fibrous capsule and supported on each side by strong collateral ligaments.

Key of abbreviations
b. Bone   **l.** Ligament
ll. Ligaments   **t.** Tendon

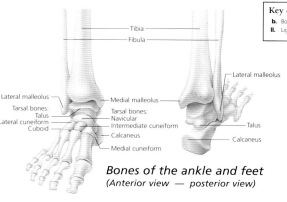

Tibia
Fibula
Lateral malleolus
Lateral malleolus
Tarsal bones:
Talus
Lateral cuneiform
Cuboid
Medial malleolus
Tarsal bones:
Navicular
Intermediate cuneiform
Calcaneus
Medial cuneiform
Talus
Calcaneus

Bones of the ankle and feet
(Anterior view — posterior view)

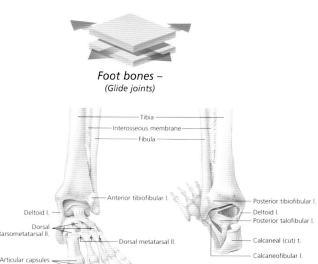

Foot bones –
(Glide joints)

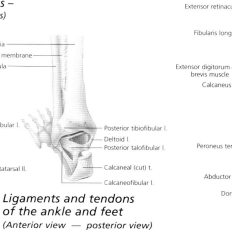

Tibia
Interosseous membrane
Fibula
Deltoid l.
Anterior tibiofibular l.
Dorsal tarsometatarsal ll.
Articular capsules
Dorsal metatarsal ll.
Posterior tibiofibular l.
Deltoid l.
Posterior talofibular l.
Calcaneal (cut) t.
Calcaneofibular l.

Ligaments and tendons of the ankle and feet
(Anterior view — posterior view)

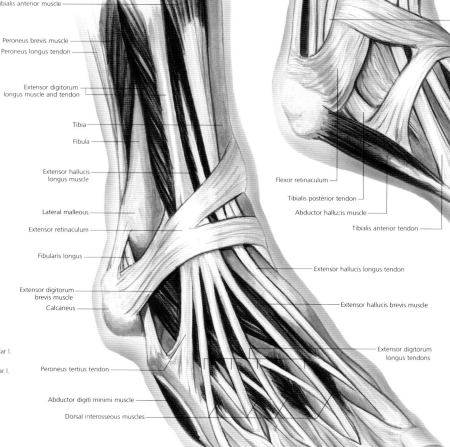

Tibialis anterior muscle
Peroneus brevis muscle
Peroneus longus tendon
Extensor digitorum longus muscle and tendon
Tibia
Fibula
Extensor hallucis longus muscle
Lateral malleous
Extensor retinaculum
Fibularis longus
Extensor digitorum brevis muscle
Calcaneus
Peroneus tertius tendon
Abductor digiti minimi muscle
Dorsal interosseous muscles
Flexor retinaculum
Tibialis posterior tendon
Abductor hallucis muscle
Extensor hallucis longus tendon
Extensor hallucis brevis muscle
Extensor digitorum longus tendons

Foot and ankle
(Anterior view)

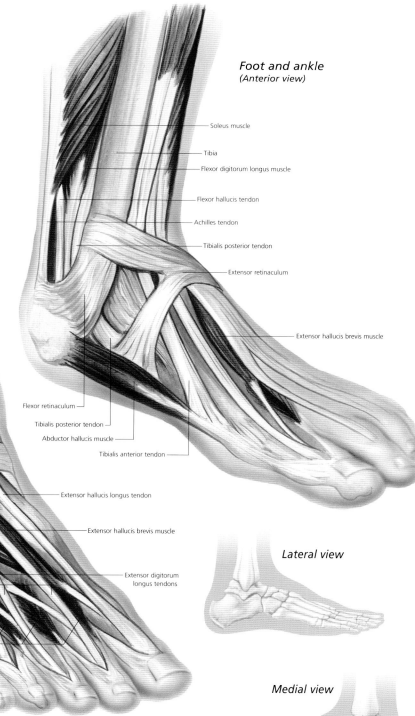

Soleus muscle
Tibia
Flexor digitorum longus muscle
Flexor hallucis tendon
Achilles tendon
Tibialis posterior tendon
Extensor retinaculum
Extensor hallucis brevis muscle
Tibialis anterior tendon

Lateral view

Medial view

Normal foot –
The longitudinal arch in the foot helps support the body as we stand or walk

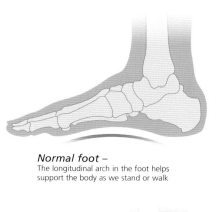

High arch foot –
Also called *pes cavus*, can be caused by muscle imbalances in the foot

Flatfoot –
Also known as *pes planus*, occurs when the longitudinal arch is gradually lost or never develops

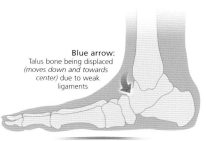

Blue arrow:
Talus bone being displaced *(moves down and towards center)* due to weak ligaments

Clubfoot –
Is a congenital deformity (present at birth) from incorrectly formed bones and joints

Bones and ligaments of the left foot
(Plantar view)

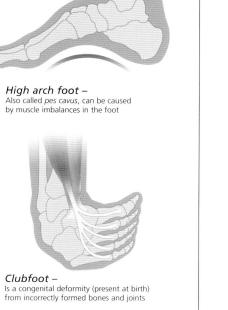
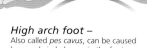
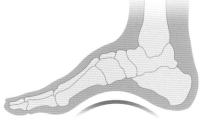
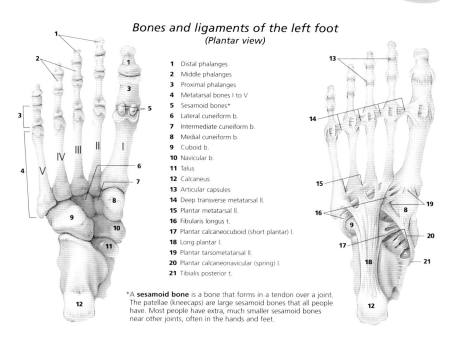

1 Distal phalanges
2 Middle phalanges
3 Proximal phalanges
4 Metatarsal bones I to V
5 Sesamoid bones*
6 Lateral cuneiform b.
7 Intermediate cuneiform b.
8 Medial cuneiform b.
9 Cuboid b.
10 Navicular b.
11 Talus
12 Calcaneus
13 Articular capsules
14 Deep transverse metatarsal ll.
15 Plantar metatarsal ll.
16 Fibularis longus t.
17 Plantar calcaneocuboid (short plantar) l.
18 Long plantar l.
19 Plantar tarsometatarsal ll.
20 Plantar calcaneonavicular (spring) l.
21 Tibialis posterior t.

*A **sesamoid bone** is a bone that forms in a tendon over a joint. The patellae (kneecaps) are large sesamoid bones that all people have. Most people have extra, much smaller sesamoid bones near other joints, often in the hands and feet.

PLATE 7

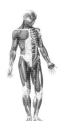

The Hand & Wrist

Anatomy of the hand and wrist

The **hand** and **wrist** together form a complex structure composed of 27 small bones connected by joints, muscles and tendons. The framework of the hand is shaped by five large **metacarpal** bones that articulate with the fingers and wrist. The fingers each contain three smaller jointed bones called **phalanges**; the thumb has two phalanges. The hand's wide range of fine movements is made possible by numerous small joints, long and short muscles, and **extensor** and **flexor** tendons that allow the fingers and thumb to straighten, bend and flex. The highly flexible thumb joint (**carpometacarpal**) is positioned at a 90-degree angle to the finger joints, giving the hand the unique ability to grasp, pinch and manipulate objects. **Tendon sheaths** surrounding the tendons contain **synovial fluid** for smooth movement of the hand and wrist.

The **wrist** connects the hand to the **ulna** and **radius** of the arm. It consists of eight **carpal** bones with multiple joints that allow flexion, extension and rotary movements. A distinctive feature of the wrist is the **carpal tunnel channel** through which the tendons from the hand pass to reach the forearm.

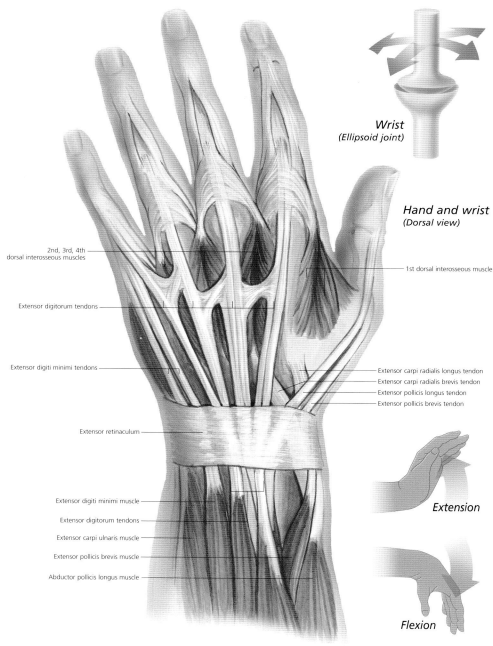

Wrist
(Ellipsoid joint)

Hand and wrist
(Dorsal view)

2nd, 3rd, 4th dorsal interosseous muscles

1st dorsal interosseous muscle

Extensor digitorum tendons

Extensor digiti minimi tendons

Extensor carpi radialis longus tendon
Extensor carpi radialis brevis tendon
Extensor pollicis longus tendon
Extensor pollicis brevis tendon

Extensor retinaculum

Extensor digiti minimi muscle
Extensor digitorum tendons
Extensor carpi ulnaris muscle
Extensor pollicis brevis muscle
Abductor pollicis longus muscle

Extension

Flexion

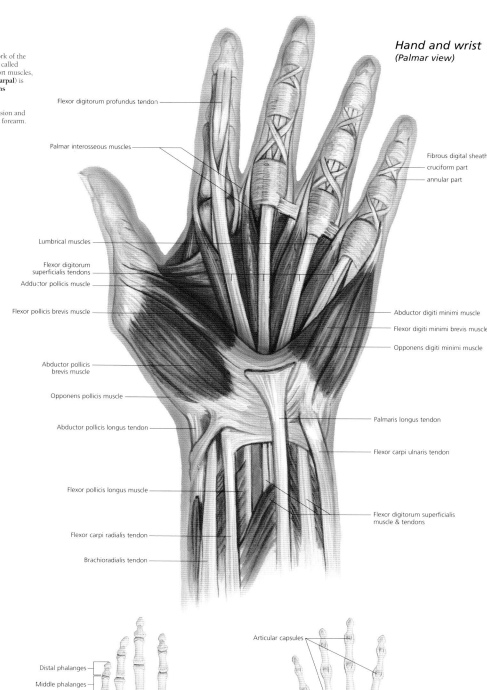

Hand and wrist
(Palmar view)

Flexor digitorum profundus tendon

Palmar interosseous muscles

Lumbrical muscles

Flexor digitorum superficialis tendons

Adductor pollicis muscle

Flexor pollicis brevis muscle

Abductor pollicis brevis muscle

Opponens pollicis muscle

Abductor pollicis longus tendon

Flexor pollicis longus muscle

Flexor carpi radialis tendon

Brachioradialis tendon

Fibrous digital sheath:
cruciform part
annular part

Abductor digiti minimi muscle
Flexor digiti minimi brevis muscle
Opponens digiti minimi muscle

Palmaris longus tendon

Flexor carpi ulnaris tendon

Flexor digitorum superficialis muscle & tendons

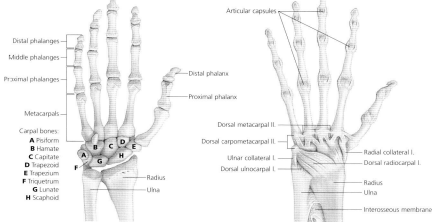

Bones and ligaments of the hand and wrist
(Palmar view)

Distal phalanges
Middle phalanges
Proximal phalanges
Metacarpals
Carpal bones:
A Pisiform
B Hamate
C Capitate
D Trapezoid
E Trapezium
F Triquetrum
G Lunate
H Scaphoid

Distal phalanx
Proximal phalanx

Radius
Ulna

Articular capsules

Dorsal metacarpal ll.
Dorsal carpometacarpal ll.
Ulnar collateral l.
Dorsal ulnocarpal l.

Radial collateral l.
Dorsal radiocarpal l.
Radius
Ulna
Interosseous membrane

Key of abbreviations
l. Ligament **ll.** Ligaments

Carpal tunnel syndrome

Carpal tunnel syndrome is an inflammatory condition affecting the median nerve and flexor tendons that pass through the **carpal tunnel**. This archway is formed by the carpal bones and sits beneath the broad **transverse ligament** extending across the palm. Inflammation and thickening of the tendons within the tunnel and the ligament above it may be caused by many factors (see right). Swelling in the tunnel compresses the median nerve, restricting blood flow and oxygen supply and causing tingling, numbness, weakness and pain in the **wrist**, **hand**, **fingers** and **thumb**. Carpal tunnel syndrome can usually be reversed if treated early. Chronic inflammation may lead to permanent nerve damage.

Potential causes of carpal tunnel syndrome include:
- Repetitive stress injuries (overuse syndrome)
- Underlying medical conditions including arthritis, diabetes and obesity
- Pregnancy
- Bone dislocations and fractures

Affected area

Sensory distribution of median nerve

Types of impairment
- Paresthesia *(abnormal sensation)*
- Hypoesthesia *(diminished sensation)*
- Anesthesia *(partial or total loss of sensation)*

Transverse carpal ligament *(flexor retinaculum)*
Palmar carpal ligament
Median nerve

(Palmar view)

Colles' fracture

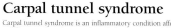

Radius
Fracture

Scaphoid fracture

Scaphoid
Fracture

Fractures

A fracture is a crack or break in a bone. There are multiple bones in the hand and wrist vulnerable to fracture, including the **carpal bones** located at the base of the hand and the **radius** and **ulna**, where they connect to the wrist.

The two most common types of fracture are Colles' and scaphoid fractures. A **Colles' fracture** is a complete transverse break in the end of the radius, and often occurs when the hand is flexed to stop a fall. It is a common injury in older people. A fall on the palm of the hand can also cause a **scaphoid fracture**, a break in the scaphoid carpal bone that articulates with the radius. This injury may initially be confused with a bad sprain and tends to heal slowly due to limited blood supply.

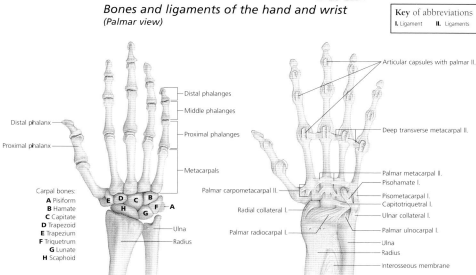

Distal phalanx
Proximal phalanx

Distal phalanges
Middle phalanges
Proximal phalanges
Metacarpals

Carpal bones:
A Pisiform
B Hamate
C Capitate
D Trapezoid
E Trapezium
F Triquetrum
G Lunate
H Scaphoid

Ulna
Radius

Articular capsules with palmar ll.

Deep transverse metacarpal ll.

Palmar metacarpal ll.
Pisohamate l.
Pisometacarpal l.
Capitotriquetral l.
Ulnar collateral l.
Palmar ulnocarpal l.
Ulna
Radius
Interosseous membrane

Palmar carpometacarpal ll.
Radial collateral l.
Palmar radiocarpal l.

Bones and ligaments of the hand and wrist
(Dorsal view)

PLATE 8

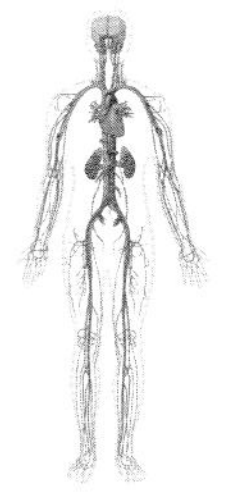

The Vascular System

What is the vascular system?

All of the parts of the body are linked by the vascular system. The system is composed of three elements: the heart, blood vessels and blood. There are three circulations involved: cardiac (through the heart), pulmonary (through the blood vessels in the lungs) and systemic (through the blood vessels in the rest of the body). Nutrients are delivered and waste products are removed from the body through the network of blood vessels in the body.

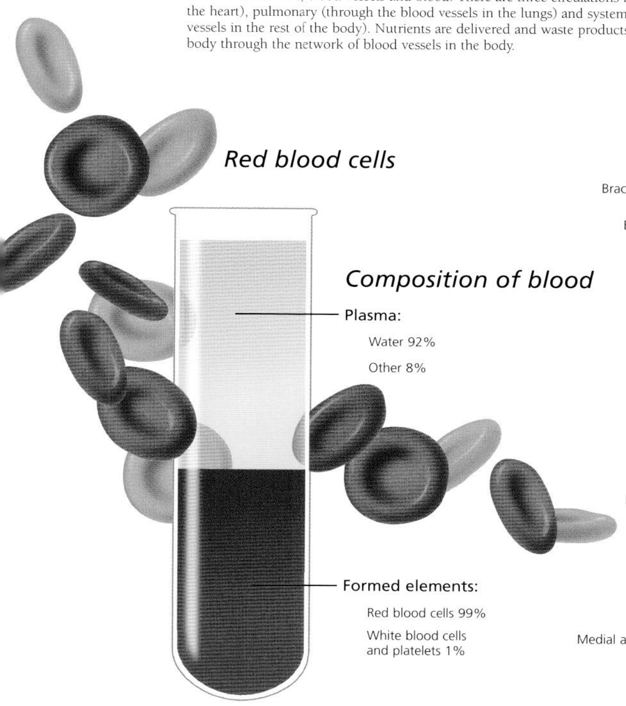

Red blood cells
Composition of blood
Plasma:
Water 92%
Other 8%
Formed elements:
Red blood cells 99%
White blood cells and platelets 1%

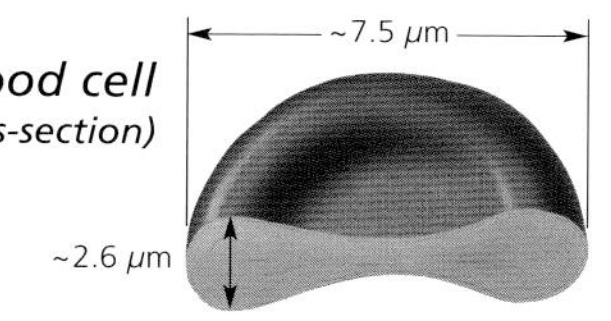

Red blood cell (cross-section)
~7.5 μm
~2.6 μm

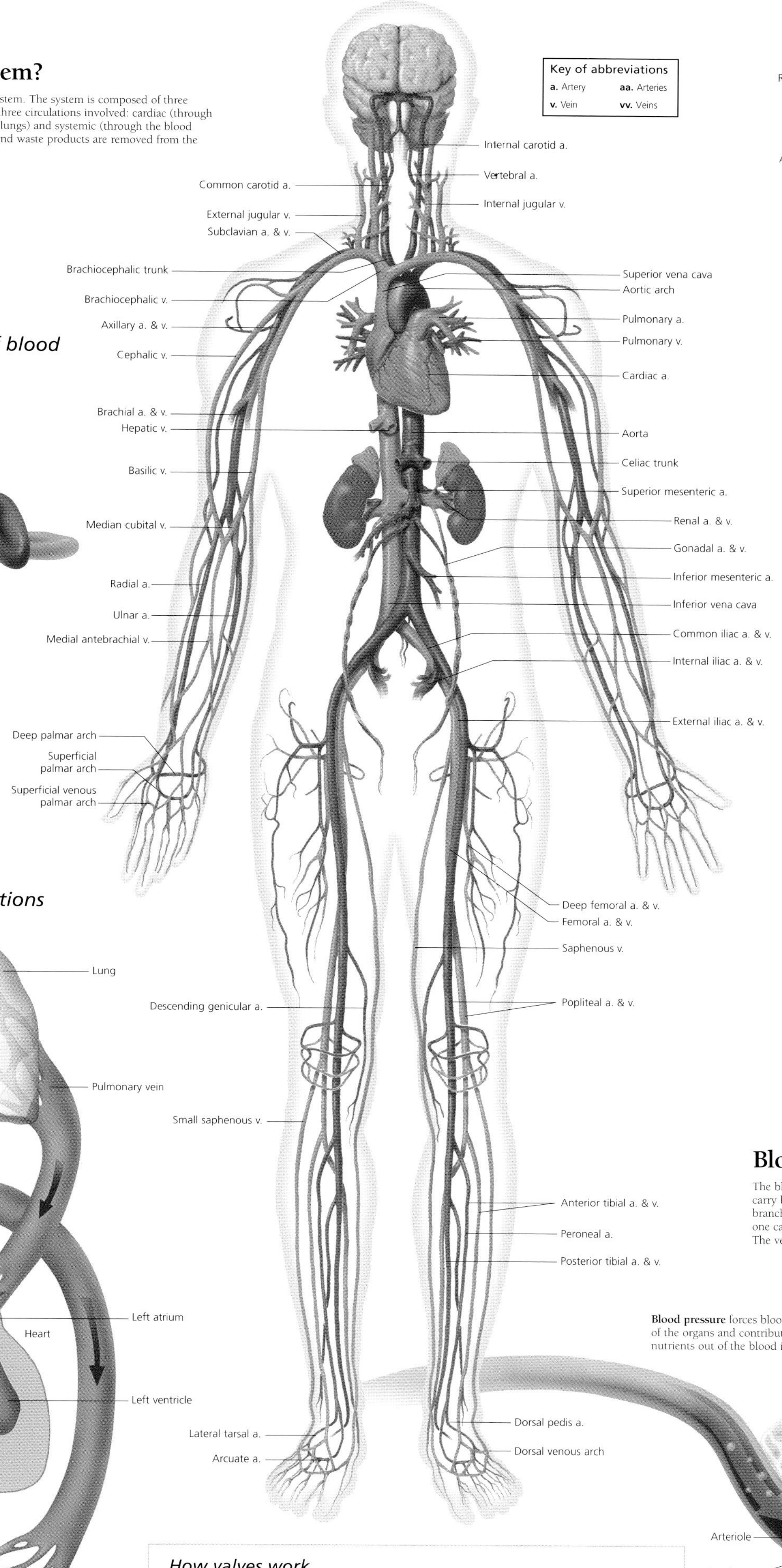

Key of abbreviations
a. Artery
aa. Arteries
v. Vein
vv. Veins
Internal carotid a.
Vertebral a.
Internal jugular v.
Common carotid a.
External jugular v.
Subclavian a. & v.
Brachiocephalic trunk
Brachiocephalic v.
Axillary a. & v.
Cephalic v.
Brachial a. & v.
Hepatic v.
Basilic v.
Median cubital v.
Radial a.
Ulnar a.
Medial antebrachial v.
Deep palmar arch
Superficial palmar arch
Superficial venous palmar arch
Superior vena cava
Aortic arch
Pulmonary a.
Pulmonary v.
Cardiac a.
Aorta
Celiac trunk
Superior mesenteric a.
Renal a. & v.
Gonadal a. & v.
Inferior mesenteric a.
Inferior vena cava
Common iliac a. & v.
Internal iliac a. & v.
External iliac a. & v.
Deep femoral a. & v.
Femoral a. & v.
Saphenous v.
Descending genicular a.
Popliteal a. & v.
Small saphenous v.
Anterior tibial a. & v.
Peroneal a.
Posterior tibial a. & v.
Lateral tarsal a.
Arcuate a.
Dorsal pedis a.
Dorsal venous arch

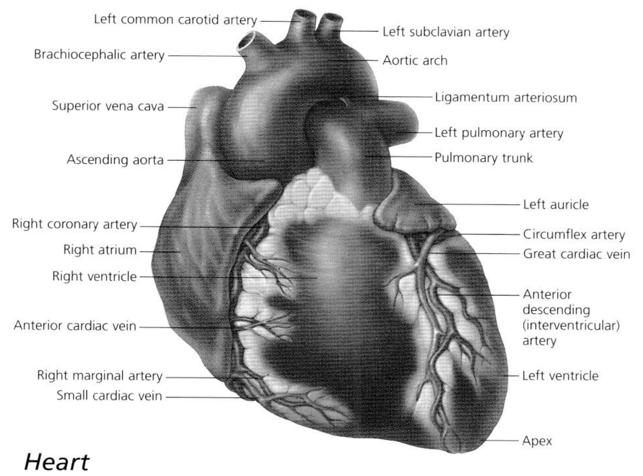

Heart
(Anterior view)
Left common carotid artery
Brachiocephalic artery
Superior vena cava
Ascending aorta
Right coronary artery
Right atrium
Right ventricle
Anterior cardiac vein
Right marginal artery
Small cardiac vein
Left subclavian artery
Aortic arch
Ligamentum arteriosum
Left pulmonary artery
Pulmonary trunk
Left auricle
Circumflex artery
Great cardiac vein
Anterior descending (interventricular) artery
Left ventricle
Apex

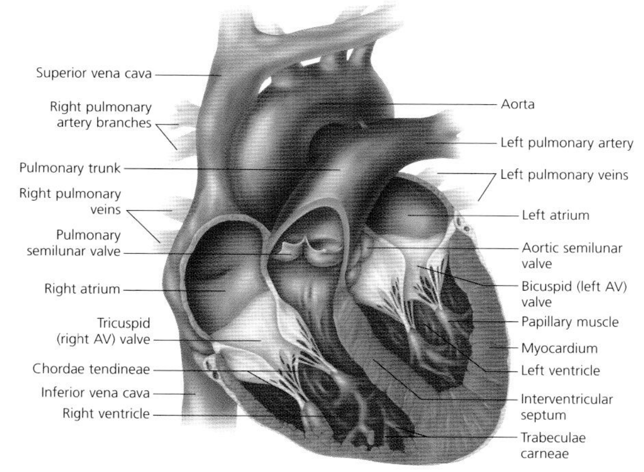

Heart
(Anterior view — partial cross-section)
Superior vena cava
Right pulmonary artery branches
Pulmonary trunk
Right pulmonary veins
Pulmonary semilunar valve
Right atrium
Tricuspid (right AV) valve
Chordae tendineae
Inferior vena cava
Right ventricle
Aorta
Left pulmonary artery
Left pulmonary veins
Left atrium
Aortic semilunar valve
Bicuspid (left AV) valve
Papillary muscle
Myocardium
Left ventricle
Interventricular septum
Trabeculae carneae

The heart

The heart is a four-chambered, muscular organ that functions as a powerful pump. About the size of a fist, the heart is located in the chest between the lungs, just to the left of center. The heart continuously pumps blood through the body's extensive network of arteries and veins. This circulation of blood delivers oxygen and nutrients to the cells while removing waste products.

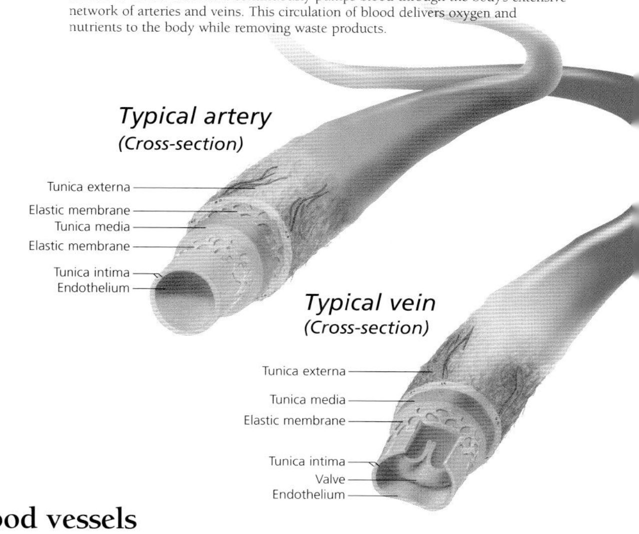

Typical artery
(Cross-section)
Tunica externa
Elastic membrane
Tunica media
Elastic membrane
Tunica intima
Endothelium
Typical vein
(Cross-section)
Tunica externa
Tunica media
Elastic membrane
Tunica intima
Valve
Endothelium

Blood vessels

The blood vessels of the vascular system include three types: arteries, capillaries and veins. **Arteries** carry blood away from the heart. The arteries branch into smaller vessels called **arterioles**, eventually branching to form a network of microscopic-sized **capillaries**. Every cell in the body is close to at least one capillary. After circulating through tissues, the capillaries merge to form small veins called **venules**. The venules merge to form **veins**, which transport blood back to the heart.

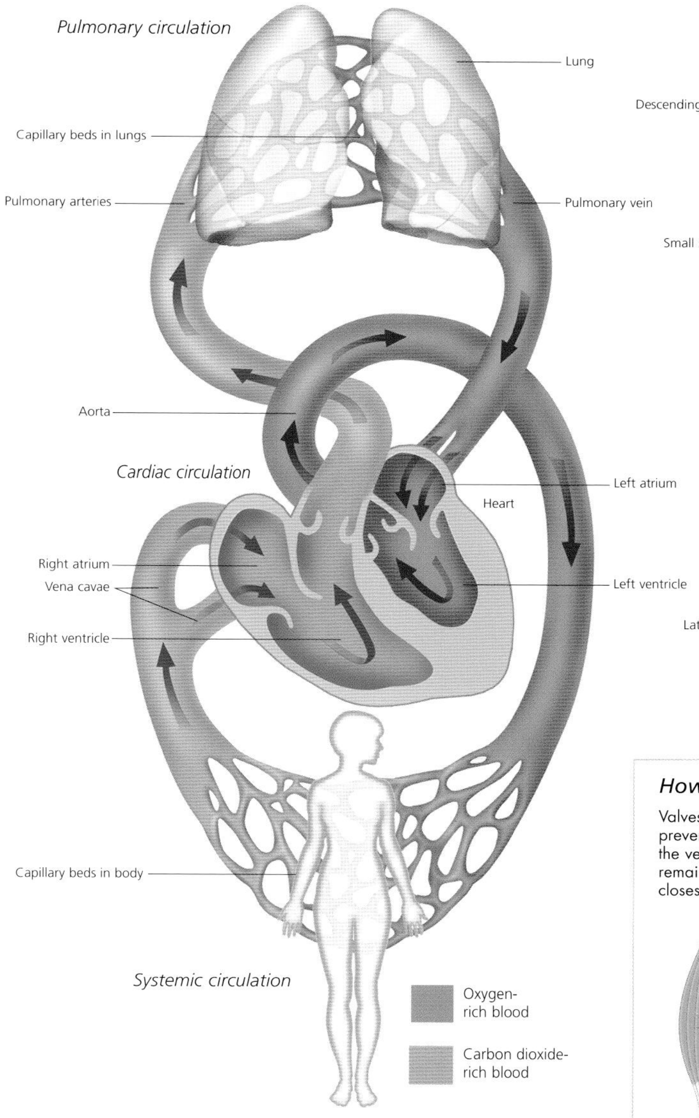

Vascular system circulations
Pulmonary circulation
Lung
Capillary beds in lungs
Pulmonary arteries
Pulmonary vein
Aorta
Cardiac circulation
Heart
Left atrium
Right atrium
Vena cavae
Right ventricle
Left ventricle
Capillary beds in body
Systemic circulation
Oxygen-rich blood
Carbon dioxide-rich blood

How valves work

Valves inside the veins open to allow blood to flow towards the heart and close to prevent it from flowing backwards. On the diagram, skeletal muscles surrounding the veins contract and compress the vein. As the upper valve opens, the lower valve remains closed, forcing the blood upward. When the muscle relaxes, the upper valve closes to prevent blood from flowing back.

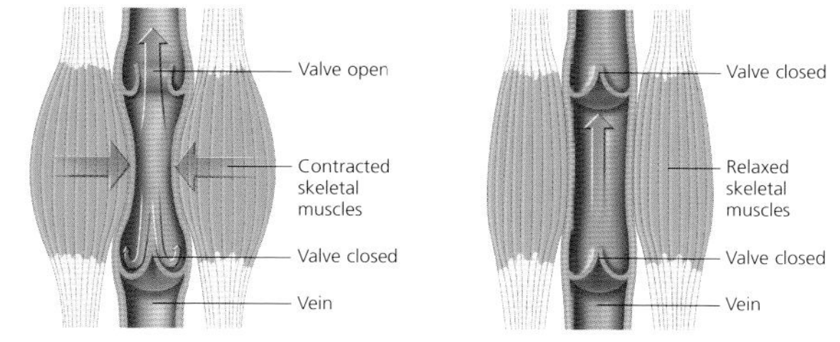

Valve open
Contracted skeletal muscles
Valve closed
Vein
Valve closed
Relaxed skeletal muscles
Valve closed
Vein

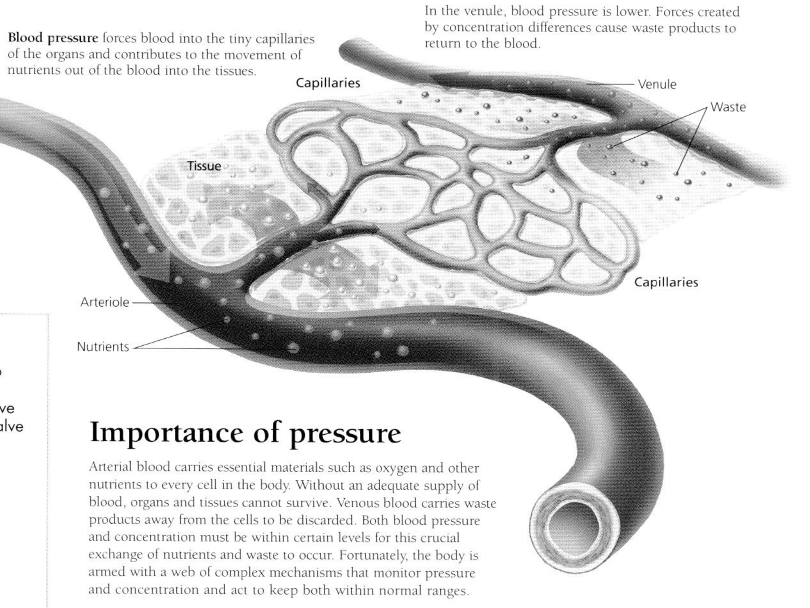

Blood pressure forces blood into the tiny capillaries of the organs and contributes to the movement of nutrients out of the blood into the tissues.
In the venule, blood pressure is lower. Forces created by concentration differences cause waste products to return to the blood.
Capillaries
Venule
Waste
Tissue
Capillaries
Arteriole
Nutrients

Importance of pressure

Arterial blood carries essential materials such as oxygen and other nutrients to every cell in the body. Without an adequate supply of blood, organs and tissues cannot survive. Venous blood carries waste products away from the cells to be discarded. Both blood pressure and concentration must be within certain levels for this crucial exchange of nutrients and waste to occur. Fortunately, the body is armed with a web of complex mechanisms that monitor pressure and concentration and act to keep both within normal ranges.

The Heart

The heart is a four-chambered, muscular organ that functions as a powerful pump. About the size of a fist, the heart is located in the chest between the lungs, just to the left of center. The heart continuously pumps blood through the body's extensive network of arteries and veins. Arteries transport blood away from the heart, and veins transport blood back to the heart. This circulation of blood delivers oxygen and nutrients to the body while removing waste products.

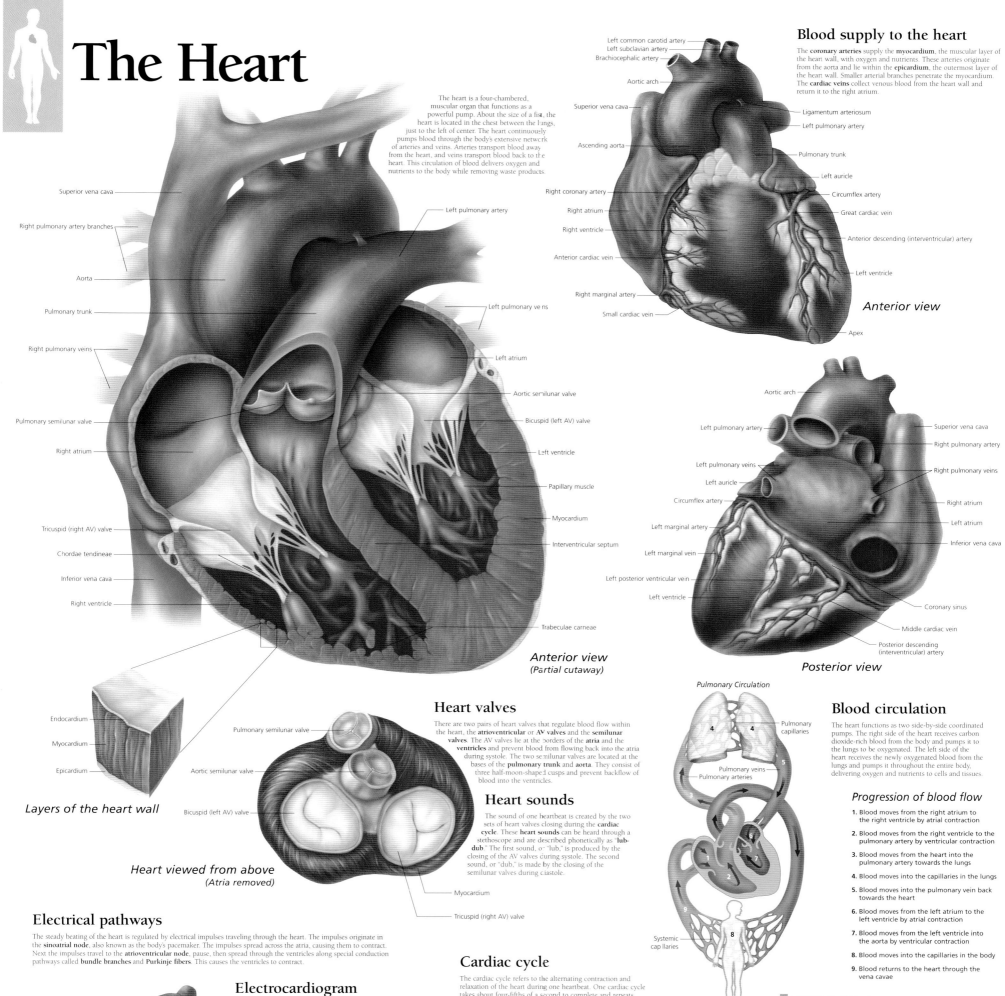

Superior vena cava
Right pulmonary artery branches
Aorta
Pulmonary trunk
Right pulmonary veins
Pulmonary semilunar valve
Right atrium
Tricuspid (right AV) valve
Chordae tendineae
Inferior vena cava
Right ventricle

Left pulmonary artery
Left pulmonary veins
Left atrium
Aortic semilunar valve
Bicuspid (left AV) valve
Left ventricle
Papillary muscle
Myocardium
Interventricular septum
Trabeculae carneae

Anterior view
(Partial cutaway)

Endocardium
Myocardium
Epicardium

Layers of the heart wall

Pulmonary semilunar valve
Aortic semilunar valve
Bicuspid (left AV) valve
Myocardium
Tricuspid (right AV) valve

Heart viewed from above
(Atria removed)

Blood supply to the heart

The **coronary arteries** supply the myocardium, the muscular layer of the heart wall, with oxygen and nutrients. These arteries originate from the aorta and lie within the **epicardium**, the outermost layer of the heart wall. Smaller arterial branches penetrate the myocardium. The **cardiac veins** collect venous blood from the heart wall and return it to the right atrium.

Left common carotid artery
Left subclavian artery
Brachiocephalic artery
Aortic arch
Superior vena cava
Ascending aorta
Right coronary artery
Right atrium
Right ventricle
Anterior cardiac vein
Right marginal artery
Small cardiac vein

Ligamentum arteriosum
Left pulmonary artery
Pulmonary trunk
Left auricle
Circumflex artery
Great cardiac vein
Anterior descending (interventricular) artery
Left ventricle
Apex

Anterior view

Aortic arch
Left pulmonary artery
Left pulmonary veins
Left auricle
Circumflex artery
Left marginal artery
Left marginal vein
Left posterior ventricular vein
Left ventricle

Superior vena cava
Right pulmonary artery
Right pulmonary veins
Right atrium
Left atrium
Inferior vena cava
Coronary sinus
Middle cardiac vein
Posterior descending (interventricular) artery

Posterior view

Heart valves

There are two pairs of heart valves that regulate blood flow within the heart, the **atrioventricular** or **AV valves** and the **semilunar valves**. The AV valves lie at the borders of the **atria** and the **ventricles** and prevent blood from flowing back into the atria during systole. The two semilunar valves are located at the bases of the **pulmonary trunk** and **aorta**. They consist of three half-moon-shaped cusps and prevent backflow of blood into the ventricles.

Heart sounds

The sound of one heartbeat is created by the two sets of heart valves closing during the **cardiac cycle**. These **heart sounds** can be heard through a stethoscope and are described phonetically as "lub-dub." The first sound, or "lub," is produced by the closing of the AV valves during systole. The second sound, or "dub," is made by the closing of the semilunar valves during diastole.

Electrical pathways

The steady beating of the heart is regulated by electrical impulses traveling through the heart. The impulses originate in the **sinoatrial node**, also known as the body's pacemaker. The impulses spread across the atria, causing them to contract. Next the impulses travel to the **atrioventricular node**, pause, then spread through the ventricles along special conduction pathways called **bundle branches** and **Purkinje fibers**. This causes the ventricles to contract.

Electrocardiogram

An **electrocardiogram** (ECG or EKG) graphically records the electrical activity of the heart. A typical ECG records three waves, each representing different phases in the **cardiac cycle**.

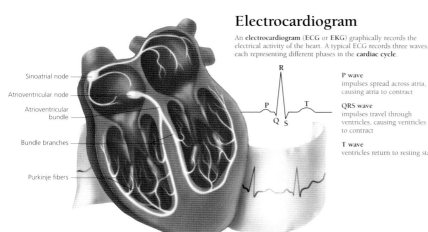

Sinoatrial node
Atrioventricular node
Atrioventricular bundle
Bundle branches
Purkinje fibers

P wave
impulses spread across atria, causing atria to contract

QRS wave
impulses travel through ventricles, causing ventricles to contract

T wave
ventricles return to resting state

Blood circulation

The heart functions as two side-by-side coordinated pumps. The right side of the heart receives carbon dioxide-rich blood from the body and pumps it to the lungs to be oxygenated. The left side of the heart receives the newly oxygenated blood from the lungs and pumps it throughout the entire body, delivering oxygen and nutrients to cells and tissues.

Pulmonary Circulation

Pulmonary capillaries
Pulmonary veins
Pulmonary arteries
Systemic capillaries

Carbon dioxide-rich blood
Oxygen-rich blood

Systemic Circulation

Progression of blood flow

1. Blood moves from the right atrium to the right ventricle by atrial contraction
2. Blood moves from the right ventricle to the pulmonary artery by ventricular contraction
3. Blood moves from the heart into the pulmonary artery towards the lungs
4. Blood moves into the capillaries in the lungs
5. Blood moves into the pulmonary vein back towards the heart
6. Blood moves from the left atrium to the left ventricle by atrial contraction
7. Blood moves from the left ventricle into the aorta by ventricular contraction
8. Blood moves into the capillaries in the body
9. Blood returns to the heart through the vena cavae

Cardiac cycle

The cardiac cycle refers to the alternating contraction and relaxation of the heart during one heartbeat. One cardiac cycle takes about four-fifths of a second to complete and repeats continuously. At rest, the heart beats an average of 60–80 times per minute. The cardiac cycle consists of two phases, **diastole** and **systole**. In diastole, the ventricles relax and fill with blood. In systole, the ventricles contract, forcing blood into the arteries.

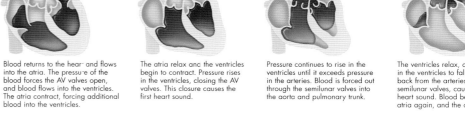
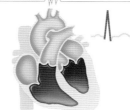
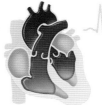
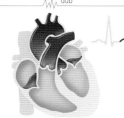

Diastole | **Systole** | **Diastole**

Heart sounds — lub — dub

Blood returns to the heart and flows into the atria. The pressure of the blood forces the AV valves open, and blood flows into the ventricles. The atria contract, forcing additional blood into the ventricles.

The atria relax and the ventricles begin to contract. Pressure rises in the ventricles, closing the AV valves. This closure causes the first heart sound.

Pressure continues to rise in the ventricles until it exceeds pressure in the arteries. Blood is forced out through the semilunar valves into the aorta and pulmonary trunk.

The ventricles relax, causing pressure in the ventricles to fall. Blood flowing back from the arteries closes the semilunar valves, causing the second heart sound. Blood begins to fill the atria again, and the cycle repeats.

PLATE 10

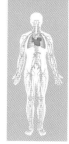

The Pulmonary System

The Pulmonary System

Inhaled air (oxygen)

Venous blood (deoxygenated)

Exhaled air (carbon dioxide)

Arterial blood (oxygenated)

What is the pulmonary system?

The pulmonary system refers to the organs of the body that cycle oxygen and carbon dioxide into and out of the lungs. Both the respiratory and circulatory systems are intricately involved in this process.

Respiration transports air to and from the **alveoli**, the functional units of the lungs. Oxygen-bearing air inhaled through the mouth and nose travels through the **trachea** (windpipe), the left and right bronchi, and into a network of progressively smaller bronchial tubes. The smallest airways, called **bronchioles**, end in microscopic **alveolar sacs** surrounded by pulmonary capillaries. This is where oxygen from the air is exchanged with carbon dioxide from the tissues and blood (see below).

Circulation functions in concert with respiration to distribute oxygen, water, and nutrients throughout the body. The circulatory system is made up of the heart, blood, and blood vessels and is divided into two pathways, pulmonary and systemic circulation.

Pulmonary circulation

The right ventricle of the heart pumps blood to the pulmonary artery, which branches into the left and right sides of the lungs. The pulmonary arteries divide and form pulmonary capillaries surrounding the alveoli. The capillaries then join together to form venules and veins, providing a pathway to return oxygenated blood to the left atrium of the heart.

Systemic circulation

Systemic circulation pumps oxygenated blood from the left ventricle of the heart (supplied by the pulmonary veins) into the aorta. From there, blood is distributed throughout the body via the arterioles and capillary networks. Systemic circulation includes all the veins carrying blood from non-lung tissue to the right atrium and all the arteries leaving the left ventricle to distribute blood to non-lung tissue.

Pulmonary circulation

- Pulmonary arteries
- Pulmonary veins

Cardiac circulation

Systemic circulation

- Veins
- Arteries

❶ Right atrium
❷ Right ventricle
❸ Left atrium
❹ Left ventricle

Cardiac circulation
How the heart works

Within the pulmonary system, the heart performs two separate but coordinated pumping actions. ❶ Blood carrying CO_2 from metabolic wastes in the body is ❷ pumped from the right side of the heart to the lungs for oxygenation. After gas exchange in the alveoli, ❸ O_2-rich blood returns to the heart to be ❹ pumped to the cells and tissues via the left ventricle, aorta and arteries.

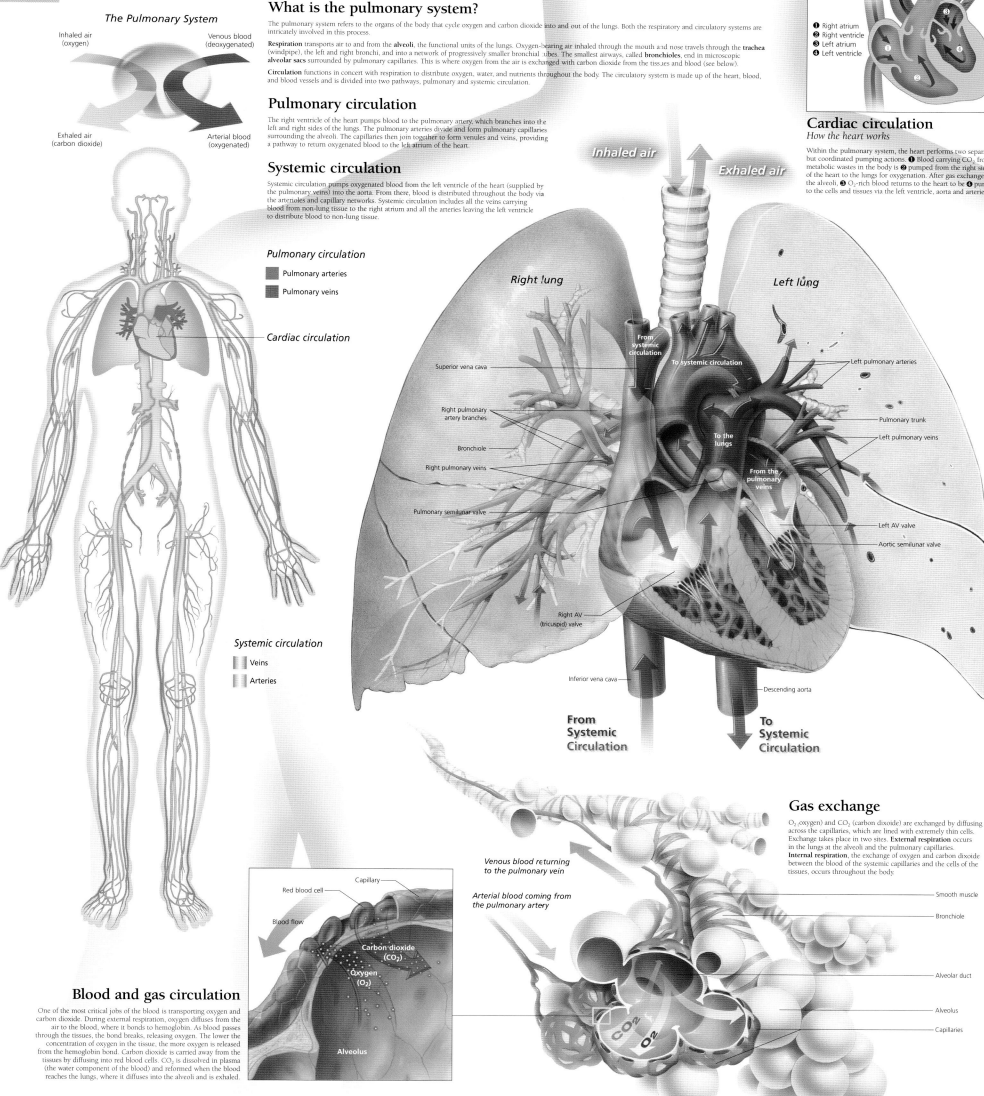

Inhaled air

Exhaled air

Right lung

Left lung

From systemic circulation

To systemic circulation

Superior vena cava

Left pulmonary arteries

Right pulmonary artery branches

To the lungs

Pulmonary trunk

Bronchiole

Left pulmonary veins

Right pulmonary veins

From the pulmonary veins

Pulmonary semilunar valve

Left AV valve

Aortic semilunar valve

Right AV (tricuspid) valve

Inferior vena cava

Descending aorta

From Systemic Circulation

To Systemic Circulation

Venous blood returning to the pulmonary vein

Arterial blood coming from the pulmonary artery

Gas exchange

O_2 (oxygen) and CO_2 (carbon dioxide) are exchanged by diffusing across the capillaries, which are lined with extremely thin cells. Exchange takes place in two sites. **External respiration** occurs in the lungs at the alveoli and the pulmonary capillaries. **Internal respiration**, the exchange of oxygen and carbon dioxide between the blood of the systemic capillaries and the cells of the tissues, occurs throughout the body.

Smooth muscle

Bronchiole

Alveolar duct

Alveolus

Capillaries

Capillary

Red blood cell

Blood flow

Carbon dioxide (CO_2)

Oxygen (O_2)

Alveolus

CO_2

O_2

Blood and gas circulation

One of the most critical jobs of the blood is transporting oxygen and carbon dioxide. During external respiration, oxygen diffuses from the air to the blood, where it bonds to hemoglobin. As blood passes through the tissues, the bond breaks, releasing oxygen. The lower the concentration of oxygen in the tissue, the more oxygen is released from the hemoglobin bond. Carbon dioxide is carried away from the tissues by diffusing into red blood cells. CO_2 is dissolved in plasma (the water component of the blood) and reformed when the blood reaches the lungs, where it diffuses into the alveoli and is exhaled.

PLATE 11

The Respiratory System

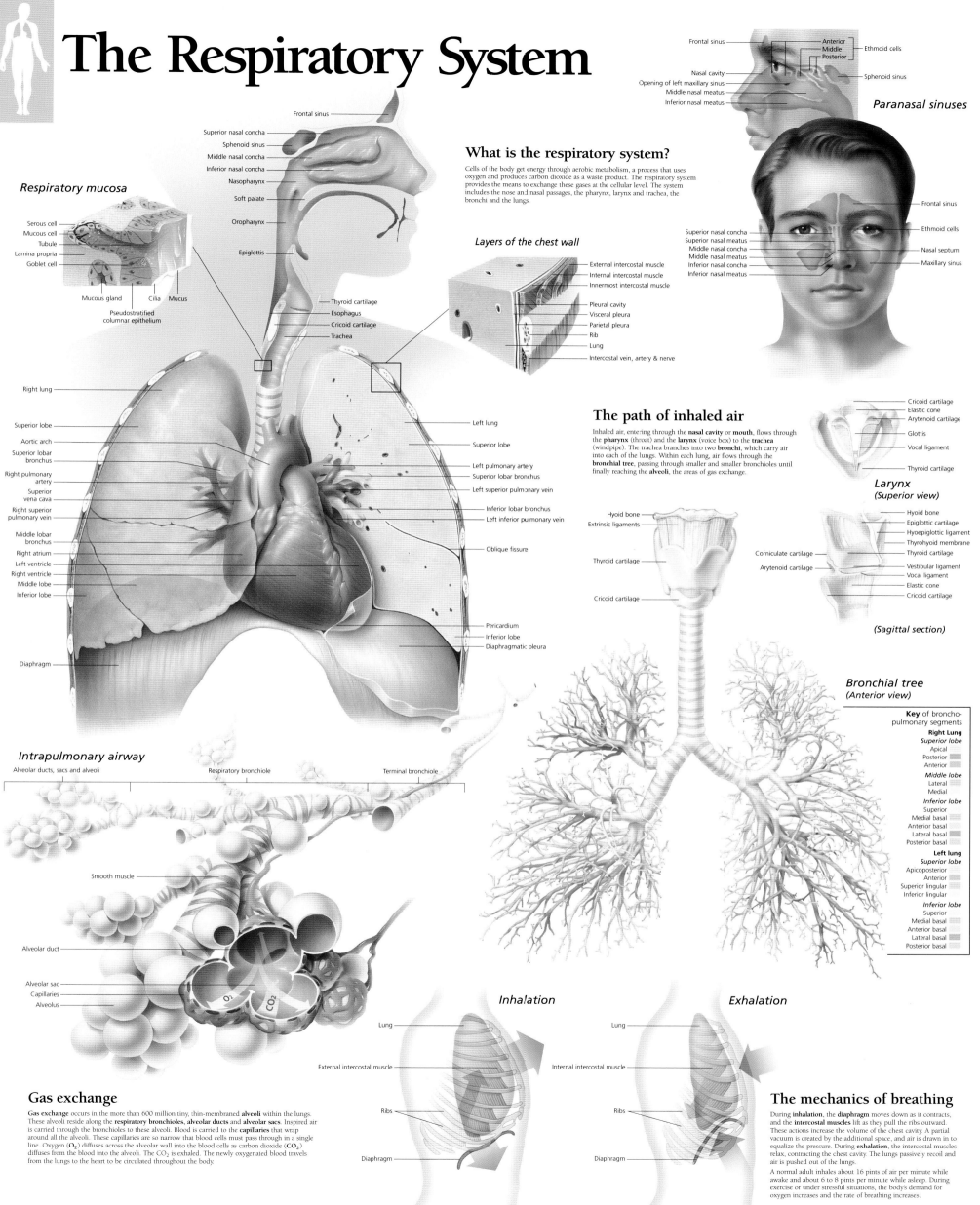

Respiratory mucosa

Serous cell
Mucous cell
Tubule
Lamina propria
Goblet cell

Mucous gland Cilia Mucus

Pseudostratified columnar epithelium

Frontal sinus
Superior nasal concha
Sphenoid sinus
Middle nasal concha
Inferior nasal concha
Nasopharynx
Soft palate
Oropharynx
Epiglottis

Thyroid cartilage
Esophagus
Cricoid cartilage
Trachea

Right lung
Superior lobe
Aortic arch
Superior lobar bronchus
Right pulmonary artery
Superior vena cava
Right superior pulmonary vein
Middle lobar bronchus
Right atrium
Left ventricle
Right ventricle
Middle lobe
Inferior lobe

Diaphragm

Left lung
Superior lobe
Left pulmonary artery
Superior lobar bronchus
Left superior pulmonary vein
Inferior lobar bronchus
Left inferior pulmonary vein

Oblique fissure

Pericardium
Inferior lobe
Diaphragmatic pleura

What is the respiratory system?

Cells of the body get energy through aerobic metabolism, a process that uses oxygen and produces carbon dioxide as a waste product. The respiratory system provides the means to exchange these gases at the cellular level. The system includes the nose and nasal passages, the pharynx, larynx and trachea, the bronchi and the lungs.

Layers of the chest wall

External intercostal muscle
Internal intercostal muscle
Innermost intercostal muscle
Pleural cavity
Visceral pleura
Parietal pleura
Rib
Lung
Intercostal vein, artery & nerve

The path of inhaled air

Inhaled air, entering through the **nasal cavity** or **mouth**, flows through the **pharynx** (throat) and the **larynx** (voice box) to the **trachea** (windpipe). The trachea branches into two **bronchi**, which carry air into each of the lungs. Within each lung, air flows through the **bronchial tree**, passing through smaller and smaller bronchioles until finally reaching the **alveoli**, the areas of gas exchange.

Frontal sinus
Nasal cavity
Opening of left maxillary sinus
Middle nasal meatus
Inferior nasal meatus

Anterior
Middle
Posterior
Ethmoid cells
Sphenoid sinus

Paranasal sinuses

Superior nasal concha
Superior nasal meatus
Middle nasal concha
Middle nasal meatus
Inferior nasal concha
Inferior nasal meatus

Frontal sinus
Ethmoid cells
Nasal septum
Maxillary sinus

Hyoid bone
Extrinsic ligaments
Thyroid cartilage
Cricoid cartilage

Cricoid cartilage
Elastic cone
Arytenoid cartilage
Glottis
Vocal ligament
Thyroid cartilage

Larynx
(Superior view)

Hyoid bone
Epiglottic cartilage
Hyoepiglottic ligament
Thyrohyoid membrane
Thyroid cartilage
Vestibular ligament
Vocal ligament
Elastic cone
Cricoid cartilage

Corniculate cartilage
Arytenoid cartilage

(Sagittal section)

Bronchial tree
(Anterior view)

Key of broncho-pulmonary segments

Right Lung
Superior lobe
Apical
Posterior
Anterior
Middle lobe
Lateral
Medial
Inferior lobe
Superior
Medial basal
Anterior basal
Lateral basal
Posterior basal

Left lung
Superior lobe
Apicoposterior
Anterior
Superior lingular
Inferior lingular
Inferior lobe
Superior
Medial basal
Anterior basal
Lateral basal
Posterior basal

Intrapulmonary airway

Alveolar ducts, sacs and alveoli
Respiratory bronchiole
Terminal bronchiole

Smooth muscle

Alveolar duct

Alveolar sac
Capillaries
Alveolus

O_2 CO_2

Inhalation

Lung
External intercostal muscle
Ribs
Diaphragm

Exhalation

Lung
Internal intercostal muscle
Ribs
Diaphragm

Gas exchange

Gas exchange occurs in the more than 600 million tiny, thin-membraned **alveoli** within the lungs. These alveoli reside along the **respiratory bronchioles, alveolar ducts** and **alveolar sacs**. Inspired air is carried through the bronchioles to these alveoli. Blood is carried to the **capillaries** that wrap around all the alveoli. These capillaries are so narrow that blood cells must pass through in a single line. Oxygen (O_2) diffuses across the alveolar wall into the blood cells as carbon dioxide (CO_2) diffuses from the blood into the alveoli. The CO_2 is exhaled. The newly oxygenated blood travels from the lungs to the heart to be circulated throughout the body.

The mechanics of breathing

During **inhalation**, the **diaphragm** moves down as it contracts, and the **intercostal muscles** lift as they pull the ribs outward. These actions increase the volume of the chest cavity. A partial vacuum is created by the additional space, and air is drawn in to equalize the pressure. During **exhalation**, the intercostal muscles relax, contracting the chest cavity. The lungs passively recoil and air is pushed out of the lungs.

A normal adult inhales about 16 pints of air per minute while awake and about 6 to 8 pints per minute while asleep. During exercise or under stressful situations, the body's demand for oxygen increases and the rate of breathing increases.

PLATE 12

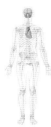

The Nervous System

The nervous system

The nervous system is composed of two integrated subdivisions that are responsible for conducting and processing sensory and motor information: the **central nervous system** (CNS) and the **peripheral nervous system** (PNS), which connects the CNS to the rest of the body.

The CNS includes the **brain** and **spinal cord**, which are covered by protective membranes called meninges (dura mater, arachnoid mater, and pia mater). The brain processes and coordinates all neural signals received from the spinal cord as well as its own nerves, such as the olfactory and optic nerves. It also performs complex mental functions such as thinking and learning.

The peripheral nervous system transmits input gathered from the sensory organs to the CNS. Motor output signals are relayed back to the PNS and on to the body's muscles and glands. The PNS has three separate divisions called the autonomic, sensory and motor nervous systems.

The functional units of the nervous system are **neurons**. **Sensory neurons** communicate information from sensory receptors to the CNS. **Motor neurons** relay signals from the CNS to effector (muscle and gland) cells. **Interneurons** coordinate and integrate sensory inputs and motor outputs. **Glial cells** also make up a significant portion of the nervous system and provide important support for neuron activity.

Spinal cord

Central canal
Anterior fissure
Gray matter
White matter
Posterior (sensory) root of spinal nerve
Denticulate ligament
Meninges:
Pia mater
Sensory root ganglion
Arachnoid mater
Dura mater
Anterior (motor) root of spinal nerve

The spinal cord and nerves

The spinal cord connects the peripheral nervous system to the brain, coordinates simple reflexes to stimuli, and helps regulate the internal organs. It contains 31 pairs of **spinal nerves**, which include both sensory and motor axons. Nerve signals generated by the sensory neurons travel through the spinal cord to the brain. Signals from the motor areas of the brain are sent back through the cord and directed to the motor neurons, triggering a response.

The inner core of the spinal cord is gray matter composed of neuron cells, glial cells, and interneurons. The outer core or white matter is made up of tracts of myelinated axons responsible for transporting nerve signals. Surrounding the spinal cord are the meninges, protective bones of the vertebral column and a cushioning layer of fat and connective tissue in the epidural space.

Dendrites
Nucleus
Cell body
Nissl bodies (produce neurotransmitters)

Direction of conduction

Structure of motor neurons

Motor neurons transmit impulses to other cells, specifically muscle fibers or glands. Each neuron consists of a **central cell body** with a nucleus and numerous fiber-like extensions called dendrites that collect and relay information to the cell body for processing. Nerve signals directed from the cell body towards target cells via the axon, a long extension of the cell membrane. An insulating **myelin sheath** made up of lipid-like **Schwann cells** insulates the axon. Spaces between these cells are called the **nodes of Ranvier**. The **axon** branches into terminal fibers which end in **presynaptic knobs** where neurotransmitter molecules are stored.

Axon
Myelin sheath (formed by Schwann cells)
Node of Ranvier

Synaptic knob or axon terminal of presynaptic neuron

Synaptic knob (or axon terminal of presynaptic neuron)
Axon terminal fiber

Mitochondria
Synaptic vesicles
Neurotransmitter molecules
Synaptic cleft
Receptor sites
Ions
Postsynaptic cell

What are synaptic connections?

Neurons in the CNS create thousands of input and output connections with other neurons, forming dense networks within the brain. Fiber-like structures called **dendrites** extend from the membrane of each neuron to receive and transmit signals from other neurons into the cell body. A long, tube-like extension called the **axon** sends signals from the neuron towards nearby target cells. As impulses arrive at the tip of the axon, the terminal bulbs release "messenger" molecules called **neurotransmitters**. These highly specialized chemicals carry nerve impulses across the tiny space between the axon and the adjacent neurons or cells, either inhibiting or activating neural impulses in the target cell.

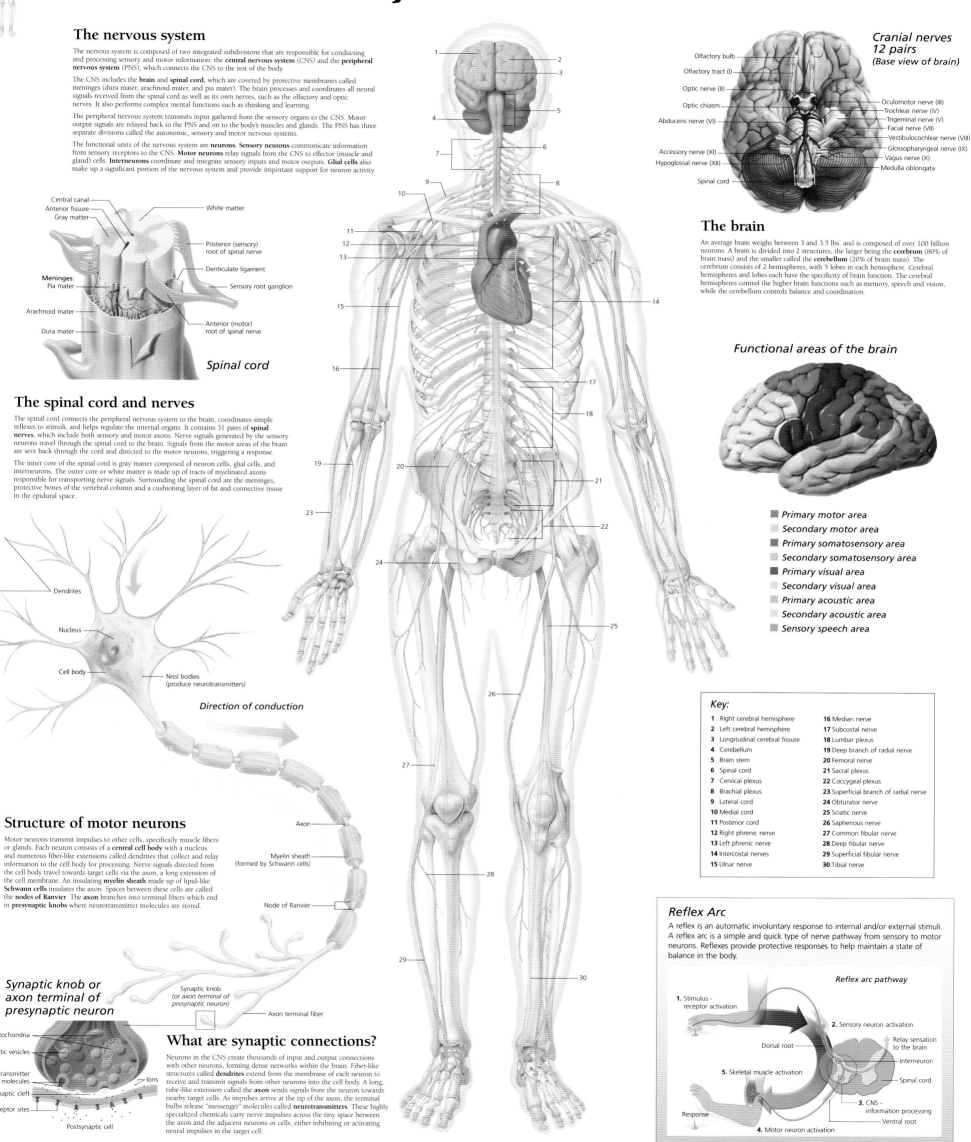

Cranial nerves 12 pairs (Base view of brain)

Olfactory bulb
Olfactory tract (I)
Optic nerve (II)
Optic chiasm
Abducens nerve (VI)
Accessory nerve (XI)
Hypoglossal nerve (XII)
Spinal cord
Oculomotor nerve (III)
Trochlear nerve (IV)
Trigeminal nerve (V)
Facial nerve (VII)
Vestibulocochlear nerve (VIII)
Glossopharyngeal nerve (IX)
Vagus nerve (X)
Medulla oblongata

The brain

An average brain weighs between 3 and 3.5 lbs. and is composed of over 100 billion neurons. A brain is divided into 2 structures, the larger being the **cerebrum** (80% of brain mass) and the smaller called the **cerebellum** (20% of brain mass). The cerebrum consists of 2 hemispheres, with 5 lobes in each hemisphere. Cerebral hemispheres and lobes each have the specificity of brain function. The cerebral hemispheres control the higher brain functions such as memory, speech and vision, while the cerebellum controls balance and coordination.

Functional areas of the brain

■ Primary motor area
□ Secondary motor area
■ Primary somatosensory area
□ Secondary somatosensory area
■ Primary visual area
□ Secondary visual area
■ Primary acoustic area
□ Secondary acoustic area
■ Sensory speech area

Key:

1 Right cerebral hemisphere	**16** Median nerve
2 Left cerebral hemisphere	**17** Subcostal nerve
3 Longitudinal cerebral fissure	**18** Lumbar plexus
4 Cerebellum	**19** Deep branch of radial nerve
5 Brain stem	**20** Femoral nerve
6 Spinal cord	**21** Sacral plexus
7 Cervical plexus	**22** Coccygeal plexus
8 Brachial plexus	**23** Superficial branch of radial nerve
9 Lateral cord	**24** Obturator nerve
10 Medial cord	**25** Sciatic nerve
11 Posterior cord	**26** Saphenous nerve
12 Right phrenic nerve	**27** Common fibular nerve
13 Left phrenic nerve	**28** Deep fibular nerve
14 Intercostal nerves	**29** Superficial fibular nerve
15 Ulnar nerve	**30** Tibial nerve

Reflex Arc

A reflex is an automatic involuntary response to internal and/or external stimuli. A reflex arc is a simple and quick type of nerve pathway from sensory to motor neurons. Reflexes provide protective responses to help maintain a state of balance in the body.

Reflex arc pathway

1. Stimulus - receptor activation
2. Sensory neuron activation
Relay sensation to the brain
Dorsal root
Interneuron
5. Skeletal muscle activation
Spinal cord
3. CNS - information processing
Response
Ventral root
4. Motor neuron activation

PLATE 13

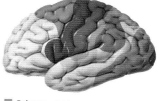

The Brain

An average brain weighs between 3 and 3.5 lbs. and is composed of over 100 billion neurons. A brain is divided into 2 structures, the largest being the **cerebrum** (80% of brain mass) and the smaller called the **cerebellum** (20% of brain mass). The cerebrum consists of 2 hemispheres with 5 lobes in each hemisphere. Cerebral hemispheres and lobes each have the specificity of brain function. The cerebral hemispheres control the higher brain functions such as memory, speech and vision, while the cerebellum controls balance and coordination. The brain accounts for about 2% of a person's body weight, yet it receives about 20% of the body's total cardiac output. Interruptions in blood flow to the brain can cause unconsciousness in as little time as 10 seconds or less.

Lobes

Key :

- Frontal lobe
- Temporal lobe
- Parietal lobe
- Occipital lobe

Limbic lobe not shown

Functional areas of the brain

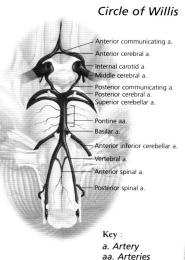

- Primary motor area
- Secondary motor area
- Primary somatosensory area
- Secondary somatosensory area
- Primary visual area
- Secondary visual area
- Primary acoustic area
- Secondary acoustic area
- Sensory speech area

Circle of Willis

Anterior communicating a.
Anterior cerebral a.
Internal carotid a.
Middle cerebral a.
Posterior communicating a.
Posterior cerebral a.
Superior cerebellar a.
Pontine aa.
Basilar a.
Anterior inferior cerebellar a.
Vertebral a.
Anterior spinal a.
Posterior spinal a.

Key :
a. Artery
aa. Arteries

Brain
(Base view)

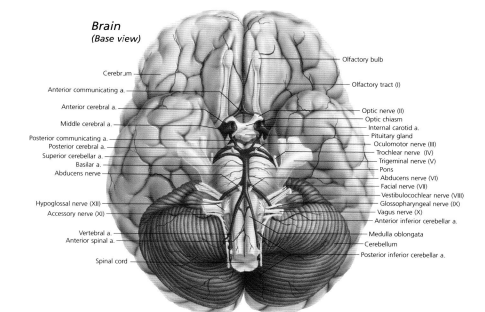

Cerebrum
Anterior communicating a.
Anterior cerebral a.
Middle cerebral a.
Posterior communicating a.
Posterior cerebral a.
Superior cerebellar a.
Basilar a.
Abducens nerve
Hypoglossal nerve (XII)
Accessory nerve (XI)
Vertebral a.
Anterior spinal a.
Spinal cord

Olfactory bulb
Olfactory tract (I)
Optic nerve (II)
Optic chiasm
Internal carotid a.
Pituitary gland
Oculomotor nerve (III)
Trochlear nerve (IV)
Trigeminal nerve (V)
Pons
Facial nerve (VII)
Abducens nerve (VI)
Vestibulocochlear nerve (VIII)
Glossopharyngeal nerve (IX)
Vagus nerve (X)
Anterior inferior cerebellar a.
Medulla oblongata
Cerebellum
Posterior inferior cerebellar a.

Meninges of the brain

Scalp
Periosteum
Bone
Epidural space
Dura mater
Subdural space
Arachnoid granulation
Superior sagittal sinus
Falx cerebri
Cerebral hemisphere

Arachnoid
Subarachnoid space
Cerebral vein
Pia mater

Coronal section

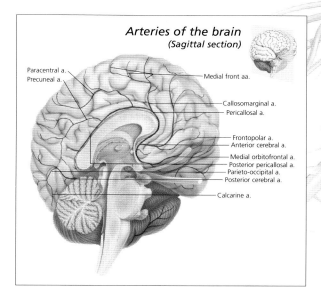

Cerebral cortex (gray matter)
White matter
Corpus callosum
Caudate nucleus
Thalamus
Hippocampus
Pons
Choroid plexus
Medulla

Lateral ventricle, anterior horn
3rd ventricle
Lateral sulcus
Lentiform nucleus
Optic tract
Interpeduncular cistern
Cerebellum

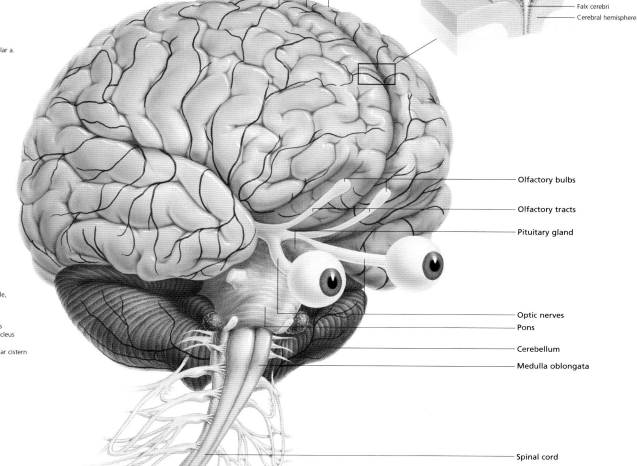

Left cerebral hemisphere
Longitudinal cerebral fissure
Right cerebral hemisphere

Olfactory bulbs
Olfactory tracts
Pituitary gland
Optic nerves
Pons
Cerebellum
Medulla oblongata
Spinal cord

Arteries of the brain
(Sagittal section)

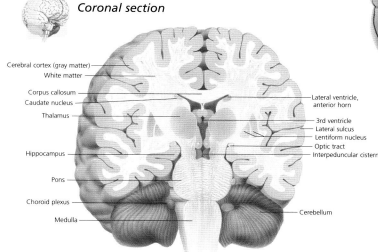

Paracentral a.
Precuneal a.
Medial front aa.
Callosomarginal a.
Pericallosal a.
Frontopolar a.
Anterior cerebral a.
Medial orbitofrontal a.
Posterior pericallosal a.
Parieto-occipital a.
Posterior cerebral a.
Calcarine a.

Limbic system
(Sagittal section)

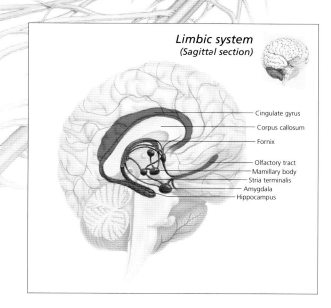

Cingulate gyrus
Corpus callosum
Fornix
Olfactory tract
Mamillary body
Stria terminalis
Amygdala
Hippocampus

Ventricles of the brain
(Lateral view)

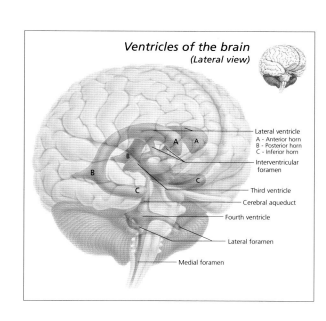

Lateral ventricle
A - Anterior horn
B - Posterior horn
C - Inferior horn
Interventricular foramen
Third ventricle
Cerebral aqueduct
Fourth ventricle
Lateral foramen
Medial foramen

A A
B
C
C

PLATE 14

The Eye

Spectrum

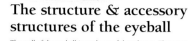

Visible Light

400nm 500nm 600nm 760nm

| Gamma rays | X rays | Ultraviolet | Infrared | Microwaves | Radio waves |

Vision

The **eye** is one of the most important of our **sensory organs**. Often referred to as "the windows to the soul", the eyes are the organs which allow us **stereoscopic vision** (depth perception), an adaptation to the environment which ensured our survival. Our eyes receive a **stimulus** from light reflected from an object and **photoreceptors** in the eye convert this light energy into nerve impulses. Only part of the **spectrum** of light, called **visible light**, can trigger these photoreceptors—wavelengths between 400 and 760 nanometers. The brain interprets these signals and gives an accurate analysis of form, light intensity, color and movement.

Labels: Eyeball, Lacrimal gland, Lacrimal duct, Iris, Sclera (covering), Pupil, Lacrimal punctum, Lacrimal canaliculi, Lacrimal sac, Nasolacrimal duct

The structure & accessory structures of the eyeball

The wall of the eyeball is made up of three layers. The outermost layer, the **fibrous tunic**, contains both the **sclera** (gives shape to the eyeball) and the **cornea** (transmits and refracts light). The middle layer, the **vascular tunic**, is made up of the **choroid** (supplies blood to the eye), the **ciliary body** (supports the lens and produces a fluid called the **aqueous humor**) and the **iris** (regulates the amount of light by controlling **pupil** size). The innermost layer, the **internal tunic**, contains the **retina** (provides photoreception and transmits impulses). Within the eyeball and suspended from the ciliary body by the **suspensory ligament** is the **lens**, which refracts and focuses the light onto the retina.

Each eye sits in a bony depression of the skull, the **orbit**, which protects and supports the eye while providing a place for attachment for the **extrinsic ocular muscles**, the six muscles that control the movement of the eye. The **eyelids** protect the eye from injury and prevent it from drying out. They distribute the fluid, called tears, that is secreted and drained by the **lacrimal apparatus**. The **eyebrows** and **eyelashes** both protect the eye from airborne and falling particles. The **conjunctiva**, a mucous membrane lining the inside of the eyelids and continuing around the front of the eyeball, prevents objects from sliding around to the back of the eye.

Scleral venous sinus

Labels: Scleral venous sinus, Cornea, Iris, Fluid movement, Lens

The **aqueous humor** produced by the **ciliary body** provides nutrients for the lens and cornea, and helps maintain the pressure in the front of the eye. Aqueous humor is reabsorbed back into the bloodstream through the **scleral venous sinus**, located at the junction of the sclera and cornea.

Right eye
(Horizontal section)

Labels: Lateral rectus muscle, Scleral venous sinus, Zonular fibers, Iris, Lens, Cornea, Pupil, Aqueous humor, Anterior chamber, Posterior chamber, Ciliary body, Sclera, Ora serrata, Conjunctiva, Choroid, Medial rectus muscle, Vitreous body, Hyaloid canal, Macula lutea, Optic disc, Retinal vessels, Optic nerve, Nerve sheath, Retina

Visual field

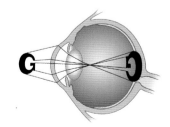

The **visual field** is the part of the external world that is projected onto the retina. The cornea and lens focus the right part of the visual field onto the left part of the retina of each eye and the left part of the visual field is focused onto the right part of the retina of each eye. Within each eye the visual field is projected upside down and reversed because of refraction.

Information about the visual field travels from the retinas to the brain. Information from the right side of the visual field travels from the left halves of both retinas to the right side of the brain. The signals from the left eye cross the **optic chiasma** to reach the right side of the brain. Information about the left side of the visual field hits the right halves of both retinas and travels to the left side of the brain—the signals from the right eye also cross at the optic chiasma. Within the brain, signals travel to areas responsible for perception and eye and body movements.

Rods & cones

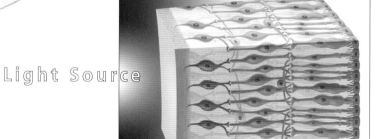

Light Source

Nerve fibers, Ganglion cells, Bipolar cells, Rods & Cones, Pigment layer

Retina
(membrane lining the back of the eye)

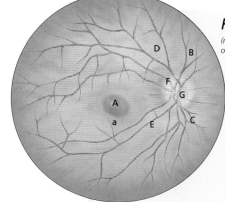

A. Fovea centralis
a. Macula lutena
B. Superior nasal artery
C. Inferior nasal artery
D. Superior nasal artery
E. Inferior nasal artery
F. Central retinal artery
G. Optic nerve

Retina

The **retina**, the internal tunic, is in the posterior part of the eyeball. It is made up of two layers, the **pigmented layer** and the **nervous layer**. The nervous layer is made of three layers of neurons: **ganglion cells**, **bipolar neurons** and **photoreceptors**. When light hits the retina, it strikes the ganglion cell layer first and then passes through the bipolar layer before reaching the photoreceptors, the **rods** and **cones**. The 120 million rods are the most sensitive to light while the 63 million cones provide color vision and greater visual acuity.

Fovea centralis

The **fovea centralis** is a small pit within the yellow area of the retina called the **macula lutea**. Visual acuity is greatest in the fovea because the area contains only cones and, due to the structure, is the only spot of the retina where light directly hits these photoreceptors.

Optic disc

The **optic disc** is where the nerve fibers from the retina gather together to exit the eye as the **optic nerve**. The disc lacks photoreceptors and is called the eye's blind spot.

Accommodation

The ability of the eye to keep an image focusing on the **retina** is called **accommodation**. When light enters the eye, it is **refracted** or focused onto the retina. In order to keep objects that are moving in focus, the eye has to adjust this refraction. It does this by changing the shape of the **lens** by use of the **ciliary body**. This muscular ring either contracts, making the lens least convex, or relaxes, making the lens more rounded or convex.

PLATE 15

The Ear

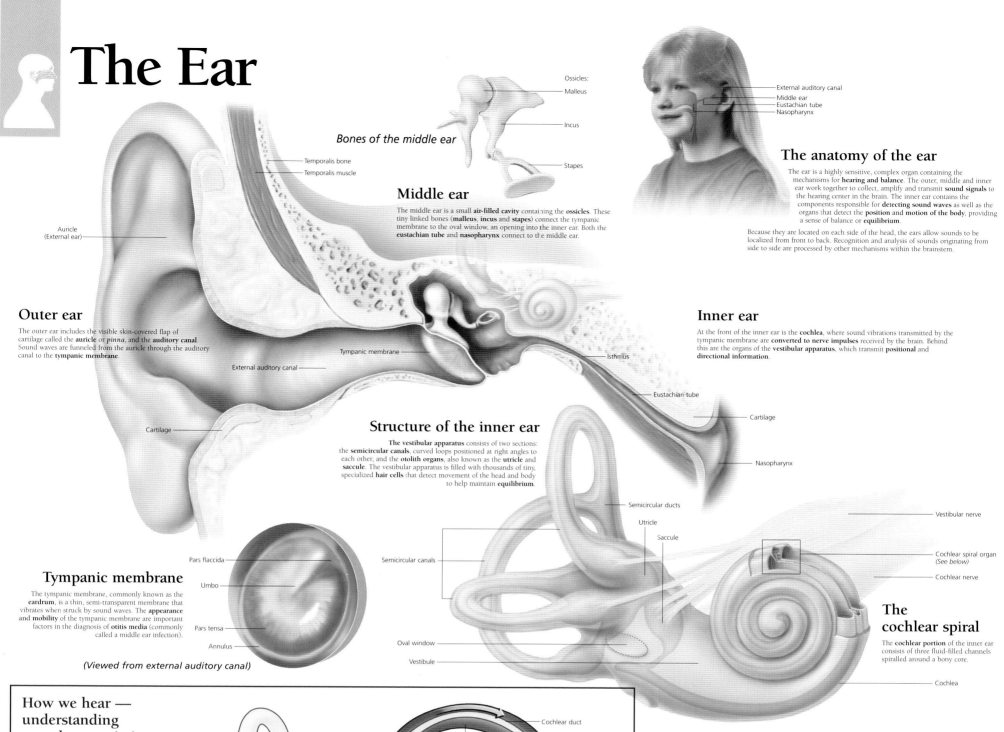

Bones of the middle ear

Ossicles:
Malleus
Incus
Stapes

Middle ear

The middle ear is a small **air-filled cavity** containing the **ossicles**. These tiny linked bones (**malleus, incus and stapes**) connect the tympanic membrane to the oval window, an opening into the inner ear. Both the **eustachian tube** and **nasopharynx** connect to the middle ear.

External auditory canal
Middle ear
Eustachian tube
Nasopharynx

The anatomy of the ear

The ear is a highly sensitive, complex organ containing the mechanisms for **hearing and balance**. The outer, middle and inner ear work together to collect, amplify and transmit **sound signals** to the hearing center in the brain. The inner ear contains the components responsible for **detecting sound waves** as well as the organs that detect the **position and motion of the body**, providing a sense of balance or **equilibrium**.

Because they are located on each side of the head, the ears allow sounds to be localized from front to back. Recognition and analysis of sounds originating from side to side are processed by other mechanisms within the brainstem.

Temporalis bone
Temporalis muscle
Auricle (External ear)

Outer ear

The outer ear includes the visible skin-covered flap of cartilage called the **auricle** or **pinna**, and the **auditory canal**. Sound waves are funneled from the auricle through the auditory canal to the **tympanic membrane**.

External auditory canal
Tympanic membrane
Isthmus
Cartilage

Inner ear

At the front of the inner ear is the **cochlea**, where sound vibrations transmitted by the tympanic membrane are **converted to nerve impulses** received by the brain. Behind this are the organs of the **vestibular apparatus**, which transmit **positional** and **directional information**.

Eustachian tube
Cartilage
Nasopharynx

Structure of the inner ear

The **vestibular apparatus** consists of two sections: the **semicircular canals**, curved loops positioned at right angles to each other, and the **otolith organs**, also known as the **utricle** and **saccule**. The vestibular apparatus is filled with thousands of tiny, specialized **hair cells** that detect movement of the head and body to help maintain **equilibrium**.

Semicircular ducts
Utricle
Saccule
Vestibular nerve
Semicircular canals
Cochlear spiral organ (See below)
Cochlear nerve

Tympanic membrane

The tympanic membrane, commonly known as the **eardrum**, is a thin, semi-transparent membrane that vibrates when struck by sound waves. The **appearance and mobility** of the tympanic membrane are important factors in the diagnosis of **otitis media** (commonly called a middle ear infection).

Pars flaccida
Umbo
Pars tensa
Annulus

(Viewed from external auditory canal)

Oval window
Vestibule

The cochlear spiral

The **cochlear portion** of the inner ear consists of three fluid-filled channels spiralled around a bony core.

Cochlea

How we hear — understanding sound transmission

Air-borne sound waves are collected by the external ear or auricle and funneled into the auditory canal, which narrows as it approaches the tympanic membrane, amplifying the waves.

The tympanic membrane vibrates in response to the sound waves and transmits vibrations to the bones of the middle ear (ossicles). Each of the three linked bones vibrates in a slightly different manner, intensifying the sound as the vibrations are carried across the air-filled cavity to the oval window, the entrance to the inner ear.

Resulting fluid pressure waves within the inner ear stimulate receptor cells in the spiral organ in the central channel of the cochlea. Nerve impulses are carried along the cochlear nerve to the auditory center of the brain and interpreted as sound.

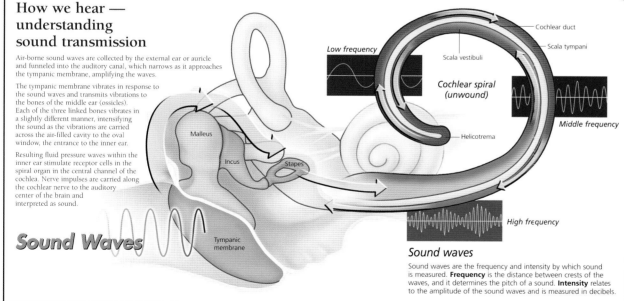

Sound Waves

Malleus
Incus
Stapes
Tympanic membrane

Low frequency
Cochlear duct
Scala tympani
Scala vestibuli
Cochlear spiral (unwound)
Middle frequency
Helicotrema
High frequency

Sound waves

Sound waves are the frequency and intensity by which sound is measured. **Frequency** is the distance between crests of the waves, and it determines the pitch of a sound. **Intensity** relates to the amplitude of the sound waves and is measured in decibels.

Cochlear spiral organ

Sound vibrations transmitted through the **tympanic** (*upper*) and **vestibular** (*lower*) canals stimulate the **spiral organ** within the central **cochlear duct**, where vibrations are converted to nerve impulses via thousands of tiny **receptor hair cells**. Adjacent nerve fibers transmit signals to the **brain stem** and **auditory cortex**.

Cochlear duct
Hair cell
Tectorial membrane
Perilymph
Hair cell
Cochlear nerve
Scala vestibuli (Lower)
Scala tympani (Upper)

Macula

The **utricle** and **saccule** each contain a sensory patch called a macula. Tiny hairs in a gelatinous mass move in response to gravity, helping to maintain **equilibrium** by monitoring the position of the head relative to the ground.

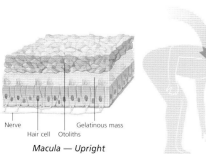

Nerve
Hair cell
Otoliths
Gelatinous mass

Macula — Upright

Gravity
Nerve
Gelatinous mass
Hair cell
Otoliths

Macula — Displaced

Understanding balance

Semicircular canals
Gravity
Utricle
Saccule
Macula sensors
Crista ampullaris sensors

The body's sense of balance or equilibrium relies on information transmitted by the vestibular apparatus, located deep within the inner ear. The **membranous labyrinth** that makes up the vestibular apparatus is filled with **endolymph** fluid, which flows in response to movement of the head and body. The fluid stimulates **tiny hair cells**, triggering sensory neurons that relay information about position and motion to the brain.

Each section within the vestibular apparatus detects and conveys specific nervous impulses.

The **semicircular canals** contain receptor structures (**ampulla**) at the base of each canal. Specialized hair cells react to changes in head position, providing **rotational acceleration** information to help the body maintain balance during spinning, tumbling or head-turning motions.

The adjacent **otolith** organs (utricle and saccule) contain sensory structures that monitor **linear acceleration**. By detecting horizontal (back and forth) as well as vertical (up and down) acceleration, these sensory cells help the body gauge how fast it is moving.

Crista ampullaris

The crista ampullaris is in the ampulla at the base of each **semicircular canal**. Sensory hair cells embedded in the cone-shaped gelatinous **cupula** respond to fluid changes in the canal during rotational movement.

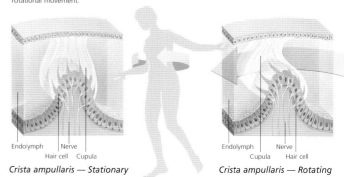

Endolymph
Nerve
Hair cell
Cupula

Crista ampullaris — Stationary

Endolymph
Nerve
Cupula
Hair cell

Crista ampullaris — Rotating

PLATE 16

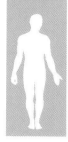

The Skin

Inside the skin

The skin is a highly elastic organ covering the entire outer surface of the body. It performs numerous functions essential to survival, including prevention of **fluid loss** from body tissues; protection against **environmental toxins and microorganisms**; reception of **heat**, **cold**, and **pain sensations**; regulation of normal **body temperature**; and maintenance of **calcium levels**.

The three basic layers within the skin are the **epidermis**, **dermis** and **subcutaneous** layers.

Epidermis. The thin uppermost layer consists of basal cells, melanocytes responsible for skin color, keratin-producing cells (for hair, nails, and outer protective skin surfaces), Langerhans cells (important in immune protection) and Merkel cells (involved in sensation).

Dermis. The dense middle layer contains the skin's structural components: nerves, blood vessels, sweat glands, hair follicles, sebaceous glands and collagen.

Subcutaneous. The underlying layer of fat cells cushions body tissues from trauma, insulates against cold and stores fuel reserves.

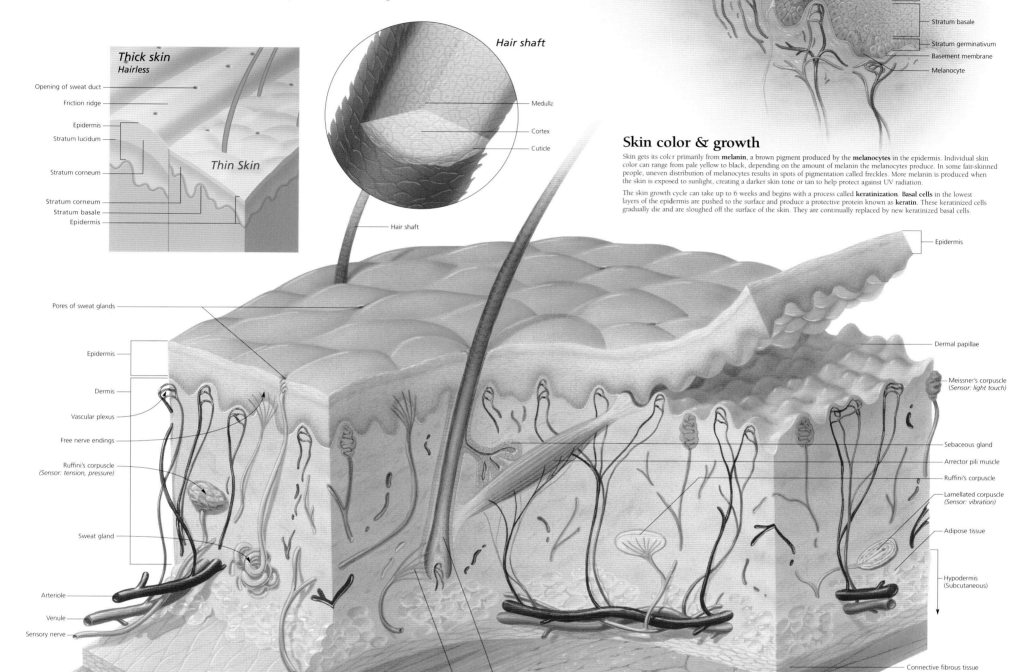

Thick skin
Hairless

- Opening of sweat duct
- Friction ridge
- Epidermis
- Stratum lucidum
- Stratum corneum
- Stratum corneum
- Stratum basale
- Epidermis

Thin Skin

Hair shaft
- Medulla
- Cortex
- Cuticle
- Hair shaft

Langerhans cell
Merkel cells
- Stratum corneum
- Stratum lucidum
- Stratum granulosum
- Stratum basale
- Stratum germinativum
- Basement membrane
- Melanocyte

Skin color & growth

Skin gets its color primarily from **melanin**, a brown pigment produced by the **melanocytes** in the epidermis. Individual skin color can range from pale yellow to black, depending on the amount of melanin the melanocytes produce. In some fair-skinned people, uneven distribution of melanocytes results in spots of pigmentation called freckles. More melanin is produced when the skin is exposed to sunlight, creating a darker skin tone or tan to help protect against UV radiation.

The skin growth cycle can take up to 6 weeks and begins with a process called **keratinization**. **Basal cells** in the lowest layers of the epidermis are pushed to the surface and produce a protective protein known as **keratin**. These keratinized cells gradually die and are sloughed off the surface of the skin. They are continually replaced by new keratinized basal cells.

- Epidermis
- Dermal papillae
- Meissner's corpuscle (Sensor: light touch)
- Sebaceous gland
- Arrector pili muscle
- Ruffini's corpuscle
- Lamellated corpuscle (Sensor: vibration)
- Adipose tissue
- Hypodermis (Subcutaneous)
- Connective fibrous tissue
- Muscle

- Pores of sweat glands
- Epidermis
- Dermis
- Vascular plexus
- Free nerve endings
- Ruffini's corpuscle (Sensor: tension, pressure)
- Sweat gland
- Arteriole
- Venule
- Sensory nerve
- Hair bulb
- Sensory receptors of hair shaft

Nail anatomy

Like the hair, nails are an accessory structure of the skin. They contain plates of densely packed, keratinized epidermal cells which arise from superficial cells in the **nail matrix**, located under the skin behind the **nail root**. Above the nail root is the visible portion of the nail, called the **nail body**. The **free edge** of the nail extends from the nail body beyond the end of the finger or toe. Near the nail root is the **cuticle** or **lunula**, shaped like a half moon.

- Nail body
- Lunula
- Eponychium
- Nail root
- Proximal nail fold
- Hyponychium
- Phalanx *Bone of fingertip*
- Epidermis
- Dermis

Warts & moles

Warts are hard, benign lumps on the surface of the skin, usually with a rough, raised surface and round or oval growth. Warts are produced when a **virus** enters the topmost layer of skin, causing an overgrowth of skin cells. Most common in children, they can be spread through **direct skin contact** and typically appear on the face, hands, or feet (often as **plantar** warts). Warts usually cause no discomfort and disappear within two years. However, treatments including medications, cryotherapy or electrocautery may be used to remove warts more quickly.

Moles are skin lesions common in light-skinned people that are often small and round and usually benign. Moles contain **melanin**, which gives them a brown or tan color. Also called **nevi** (singular: nevus), moles can range in size from tiny to very large and may have smooth or irregular borders. Unusual changes in the size or appearance of a nevus can be an important warning sign of **melanoma** (skin cancer).

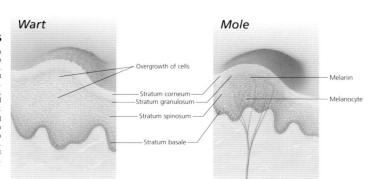

Wart
- Overgrowth of cells
- Stratum corneum
- Stratum granulosum
- Stratum spinosum
- Stratum basale

Mole
- Melanin
- Melanocyte

How we sweat

The skin contains two types of glands that produce perspiration. **Eccrine** glands, which are distributed throughout the body, open into sweat pores on the surface of the skin. In response to increased body temperature, sweat is produced in the deep coiled portion of the eccrine gland, then passes through the duct to the epidermis. It consists of water, salt and other chemicals and evaporates on the skin surface, helping to cool the body. The more specialized **apocrine** sweat glands are concentrated in the armpit and genital area and produce a thicker, oily secretion (which includes pheromones), often in response to emotional stress ("cold sweat").

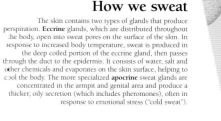
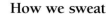

- Heat
- Sweat
- Opening of sweat duct
- Sweat duct

PLATE 17

The Digestive System

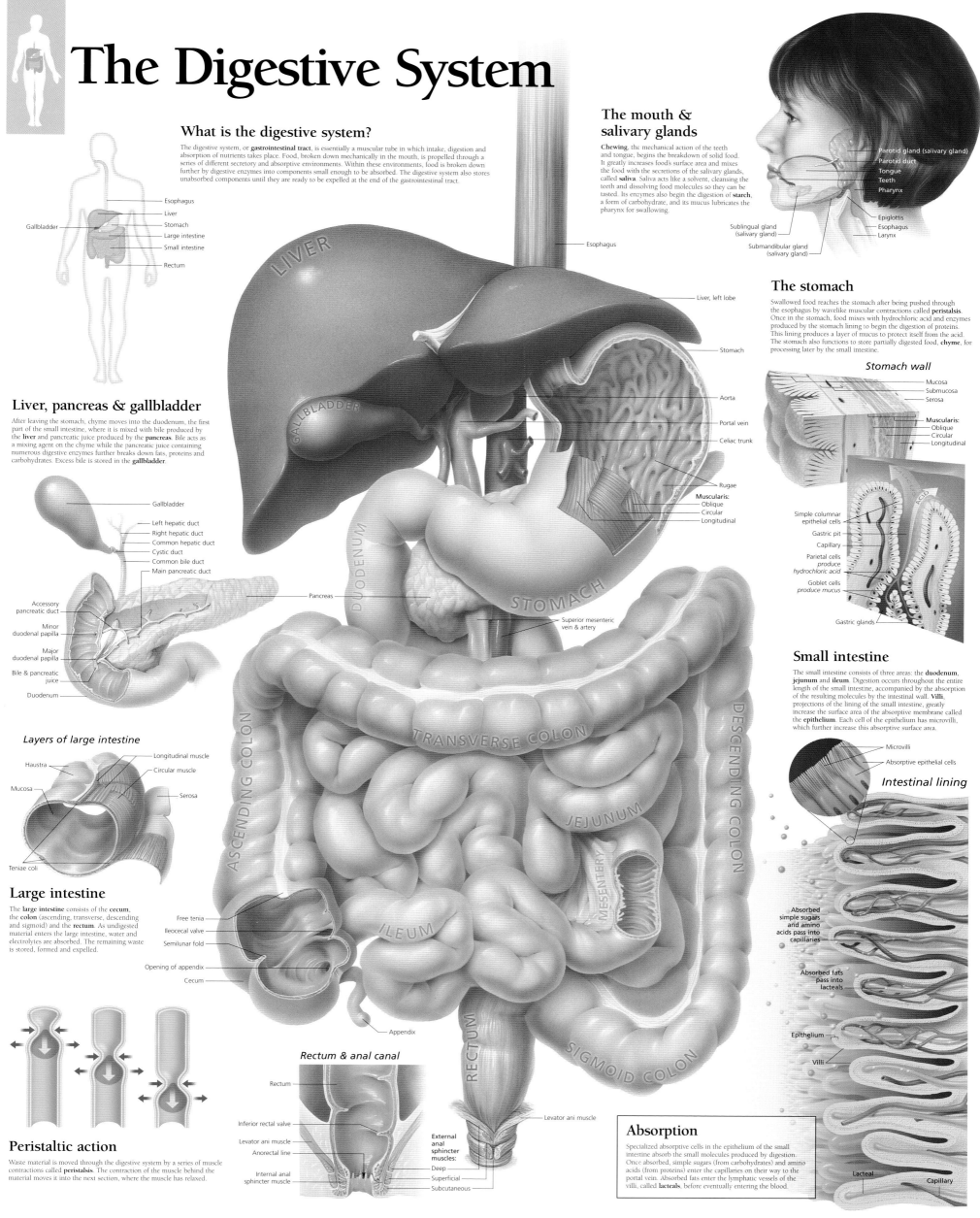

What is the digestive system?

The digestive system, or **gastrointestinal tract**, is essentially a muscular tube in which intake, digestion and absorption of nutrients takes place. Food, broken down mechanically in the mouth, is propelled through a series of different secretory and absorptive environments. Within these environments, food is broken down further by digestive enzymes into components small enough to be absorbed. The digestive system also stores unabsorbed components until they are ready to be expelled at the end of the gastrointestinal tract.

- Esophagus
- Liver
- Stomach
- Large intestine
- Small intestine
- Rectum

Gallbladder

The mouth & salivary glands

Chewing, the mechanical action of the teeth and tongue, begins the breakdown of solid food. It greatly increases food's surface area and mixes the food with the secretions of the salivary glands, called **saliva**. Saliva acts like a solvent, cleansing the teeth and dissolving food molecules so they can be tasted. Its enzymes also begin the digestion of **starch**, a form of carbohydrate, and its mucus lubricates the pharynx for swallowing.

- Parotid gland (salivary gland)
- Parotid duct
- Tongue
- Teeth
- Pharynx
- Epiglottis
- Esophagus
- Larynx
- Sublingual gland (salivary gland)
- Submandibular gland (salivary gland)

Esophagus

The stomach

Swallowed food reaches the stomach after being pushed through the esophagus by wavelike muscular contractions called **peristalsis**. Once in the stomach, food mixes with hydrochloric acid and enzymes produced by the stomach lining to begin the digestion of proteins. This lining produces a layer of mucus to protect itself from the acid. The stomach also functions to store partially digested food, **chyme**, for processing later by the small intestine.

Liver, left lobe

Stomach

Aorta

Portal vein

Celiac trunk

Rugae

Muscularis:
- Oblique
- Circular
- Longitudinal

Stomach wall

- Mucosa
- Submucosa
- Serosa
- **Muscularis:**
  - Oblique
  - Circular
  - Longitudinal
- Simple columnar epithelial cells
- Gastric pit
- Capillary
- Parietal cells *produce hydrochloric acid*
- Goblet cells *produce mucus*
- Gastric glands

Liver, pancreas & gallbladder

After leaving the stomach, chyme moves into the duodenum, the first part of the small intestine, where it is mixed with bile produced by the **liver** and pancreatic juice produced by the **pancreas**. Bile acts as a mixing agent on the chyme while the pancreatic juice containing numerous digestive enzymes further breaks down fats, proteins and carbohydrates. Excess bile is stored in the **gallbladder**.

- Gallbladder
- Left hepatic duct
- Right hepatic duct
- Common hepatic duct
- Cystic duct
- Common bile duct
- Main pancreatic duct
- Accessory pancreatic duct
- Minor duodenal papilla
- Major duodenal papilla
- Bile & pancreatic juice
- Duodenum

Pancreas

Superior mesenteric vein & artery

Small intestine

The small intestine consists of three areas: the **duodenum**, **jejunum** and **ileum**. Digestion occurs throughout the entire length of the small intestine, accompanied by the absorption of the resulting molecules by the intestinal wall. **Villi**, projections of the lining of the small intestine, greatly increase the surface area of the absorptive membrane called the **epithelium**. Each cell of the epithelium has microvilli, which further increase this absorptive surface area.

- Microvilli
- Absorptive epithelial cells

Intestinal lining

- Absorbed simple sugars and amino acids pass into capillaries
- Absorbed fats pass into lacteals
- Epithelium
- Villi

Layers of large intestine

- Longitudinal muscle
- Circular muscle
- Serosa
- Haustra
- Mucosa
- Teniae coli

Large intestine

The **large intestine** consists of the cecum, the **colon** (ascending, transverse, descending and sigmoid) and the **rectum**. As undigested material enters the large intestine, water and electrolytes are absorbed. The remaining waste is stored, formed and expelled.

- Free tenia
- Ileocecal valve
- Semilunar fold
- Opening of appendix
- Cecum
- Appendix

Peristaltic action

Waste material is moved through the digestive system by a series of muscle contractions called **peristalsis**. The contraction of the muscle behind the material moves it into the next section, where the muscle has relaxed.

Rectum & anal canal

- Rectum
- Inferior rectal valve
- Levator ani muscle
- Anorectal line
- Internal anal sphincter muscle
- **External anal sphincter muscles:**
  - Deep
  - Superficial
  - Subcutaneous
- Levator ani muscle

Absorption

Specialized absorptive cells in the epithelium of the small intestine absorb the small molecules produced by digestion. Once absorbed, simple sugars (from carbohydrates) and amino acids (from proteins) enter the capillaries on their way to the portal vein. Absorbed fats enter the lymphatic vessels of the villi, called **lacteals**, before eventually entering the blood.

- Lacteal
- Capillary

PLATE 18

The Teeth

The anatomy of the teeth

The teeth are living, calcified structures embedded in the upper (**maxillary**) and lower (**mandibular**) arches of the jaw. The part of the tooth visible above the gumline is called the **crown**. Below the gumline is the **root**, which extends into the bony portion of the jaw. The teeth are tightly surrounded by soft tissue called the **gingiva** (gums) and cushioned by shock-resistant **periodontal membrane**, which lines the bony sockets within the jaw.

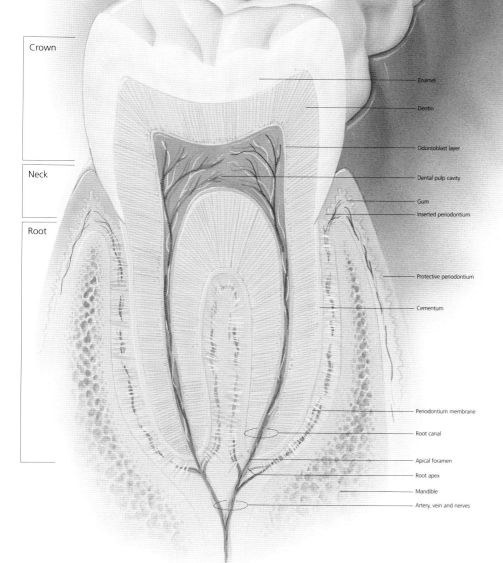

Crown

- Enamel
- Dentin
- Odontoblast layer
- Dental pulp cavity
- Gum
- Inserted periodontium

Neck

Root

- Protective periodontium
- Cementum
- Periodontium membrane
- Root canal
- Apical foramen
- Root apex
- Mandible
- Artery, vein and nerves

Deciduous dentition

Deciduous (baby) teeth are the first, temporary set of teeth. Beginning with the lower incisors, deciduous teeth typically erupt between the ages of 6 and 24 months. There are 20 deciduous teeth (10 upper and 10 lower), which remain in place until they are shed and replaced by the permanent (adult) teeth beginning around age 6, during a process known as **exfoliation**. By age 13, baby teeth are usually completely replaced by permanent teeth.

Healthy baby teeth play a key role in a child's ability to form clear speech, chew efficiently and develop normal jaw structure and facial characteristics. Extensive decay or tooth loss can have lasting effects on the appearance and development of the child's permanent teeth.

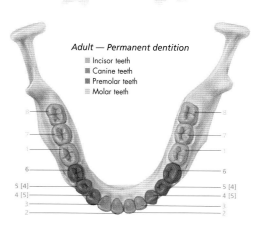

Permanent teeth

A tooth consists of four layers

Enamel is the white, highly calcified outer layer. It is the hardest substance in the body and highly resistant to acids and other corrosive agents. Enamel is without feeling.

Dentin is a hard, yellow layer of tissue beneath the enamel that forms the bulk of the crown. It is softer than enamel and transmits sensations such as temperature and pain to the root.

Cementum is a thin, bony layer covering the root portion of the tooth. It is connected to the jaw bone by collagen fibers that pass through the periodontal membrane to hold the tooth in place.

Pulp is the soft tissue in the inner cavity of the tooth. It contains the nerve fibers and blood vessels and supplies nutrients to the tooth. Pulp extends into the jaw bone and is highly sensitive to pain and temperature.

Sequence of eruption — Age of eruption (in months)

- 1 — 6 to 8
- 2 — 8 to 12
- 4 — 15 to 20
- 3 — 12 to 16
- 5 — 20 to 40

Sequence of eruption — Age of eruption (in years)

- 2 — 6 to 9
- 1 — 7 to 10
- 5 — 10 to 14
- 4 — 9 to 13
- 6 — 10 to 14
- 7 — 12 to 30

Child — Deciduous dentition

- ▪ Deciduous incisor teeth
- ▪ Deciduous canine teeth
- ▪ Deciduous premolar teeth

- 5 — 20 to 40
- 3 — 12 to 16
- 4 — 15 to 20
- 2 — 8 to 12
- 1 — 6 to 8

Adult — Permanent dentition

- ▪ Incisor teeth
- ▪ Canine teeth
- ▪ Premolar teeth
- ▪ Molar teeth

- 8
- 7
- 1
- 6
- 5 [4]
- 4 [5]
- 3
- 2

Types and functions of teeth

The adult jaw holds **32 permanent teeth** arranged in an arch, with 16 teeth on the upper jaw and 16 teeth on the lower. The general positions of the teeth within the mouth are noted as either anterior (towards the front) or posterior (towards the back). There are four types of permanent teeth:

ANTERIOR

Incisors
- ▪ Sharp, chiseled shape
- ▪ Located at the center front of the mouth
- ▪ Used to cut or shear food
- ▪ 2 central upper/lower, 2 lateral upper/lower

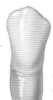

Canines
- ▪ Also called cuspids
- ▪ Shaped like points
- ▪ Work with the incisors to tear food
- ▪ Support the lips and guide jaw alignment
- ▪ 2 upper, 2 lower

POSTERIOR

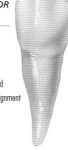

Premolars
- ▪ Also called bicuspids
- ▪ Broad surfaces with pointed cusps
- ▪ Used to crush and tear food
- ▪ Support vertical dimension of the jaw and face
- ▪ 4 upper, 4 lower

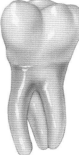

Molars
- ▪ Broad surfaces with several cusps
- ▪ Important for grinding food
- ▪ Work with premolars to maintain vertical dimension
- ▪ 6 upper, 6 lower

Impaction

Teeth become impacted when they remain embedded in the gum (**gingiva**) or bone and either fail to emerge or emerge only partially. Impaction occurs when a tooth is blocked by other teeth, because the jaw is too small or if teeth become tilted or twisted as they emerge. The most common type of impaction is in the wisdom teeth, or third molars. Symptoms may include pain in the gum or jaw, inflammation in the gum around the tooth caused by trapped debris (**pericoronitis**) and prolonged headache or jaw ache. Pressure from impacted teeth may also cause misalignment in nearby teeth. Extraction is usually recommended for symptomatic impactions.

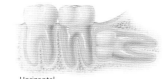

Horizontal

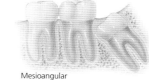

Mesioangular

Why do teeth hurt?

Pain either in one tooth or in the teeth and gums generally can occur as a sharp twinge or a dull throb.

Tooth pain during or after eating or in response to hot or cold temperatures may be caused by tooth decay, gingivitis or linked to recent dental work

Repeated episodes of throbbing pain are usually associated with advanced tooth decay/inflammation of the pulp (pulpitis)

Continuous pain and/or elevated temperature result from severe pulpitis or an abscess in the pulp or root canal

Occlusion

The alignment of the upper and lower jaws and surfaces of the teeth is called occlusion (or **bite**). In many people, occlusion abnormalities (**malocclusion**) occur as a result of disproportionate teeth and jaw size, extra teeth, tooth loss, trauma and other factors. Surgery and/or **orthodontic treatment** may be necessary to reposition and align the teeth.

Types of malocclusion Type 1: **Overcrowding** or poor positioning of the teeth. Type 2: **Underbite** (protruding lower jaw and teeth). Type 3: **Overbite** (upper jaw overlapping the lower).

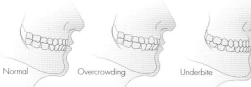

Normal   Overcrowding   Underbite   Overbite

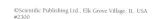

PLATE 19

The Liver

The liver weighs approximately 3 lbs. and is the largest internal organ in the body. It is located in the upper right section of the abdomen, behind the rib cage and above the stomach, right kidney and intestines. The liver is divided by connective tissue called the **falciform ligament** into two major lobes. The larger right lobe is approximately six times larger than the smaller left lobe. Two smaller lobes, the quadrate and the caudate, are located on the visceral surface.

The liver performs more than 500 important functions, including its vital role as an entry into the digestive tract and the circulatory system. It is also an important source of **blood storage**.

Approximately 1500 ml of blood flows through the liver per minute. As much as 13 percent of the body's total blood volume is usually contained in the liver, which can swell to hold even larger amounts of blood in response to injury or illness.

The portal system

The hepatic portal system is comprised of a network of veins that transport blood from the internal abdominal organs (stomach, intestine, spleen and pancreas) to the liver. Portal blood contains both **nutrients** and **toxins** that drain directly from the digestive system and must be screened before returning to the body. Specialized macrophages lining the **hepatic sinusoids** called **Kupffer cells** perform this task by detoxifying harmful substances in the blood, destroying old and defective red blood cells, and eliminating bacteria and debris. They also remove nutrients, amino acids and glucose, which are then metabolized by enzymes in the **hepatocytes**, cells that make up most of the liver's structure.

Functions of the liver

The liver is involved in many of the body's metabolic functions, including:

- Production and excretion of bile and cholesterol
- Detoxification of drugs and other harmful substances
- Metabolism of nutrients (fats, carbohydrates and proteins)
- Conversion of excess glucose into glycogen for storage
- Regulation of amino acid levels
- Storage of blood and vitamins including Vitamins A, D, E and K
- Synthesis of plasma proteins and blood clotting factors
- Conversion of ammonia to urea for elimination by the kidneys

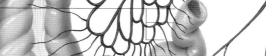

■ **Venous blood** *(filtered)*
■ **Portal blood** *(unfiltered)*

To Heart — Esophagus
Inferior vena cava
Liver
Hepatic portal vein
Gastric vein
Splenic vein
Spleen
Stomach
Superior mesenteric v.
Right colic vein
Inferior mesenteric vein
Intestinal veins
Appendix

Bile production

A major digestive function of the liver is the production of **bile**, a combination of water, bile salts, bile pigments, phospholipids, cholesterol and other substances. Bile is used during digestion to neutralize stomach acids and emulsify (break down) fats in the duodenum, which is attached to the stomach and forms the upper segment of the small intestine. Bile is produced by the **hepatocytes** and secreted into the bile channels for storage in the **gallbladder**, a small, pear-shaped organ on the visceral surface of the liver. Much of the bile used in digestion is **reabsorbed** by the small intestine and later returned to the liver.

Bile secretion is stimulated by a hormone secretin. Bile exits the liver via the right and left hepatic ducts, which join to form a common hepatic duct. This combines with the cystic duct from the gallbladder, creating the common bile duct. Bile travels along the common bile duct to join the pancreatic duct at the duodenum.

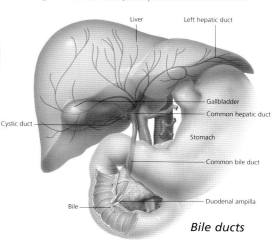

Liver — Left hepatic duct
Gallbladder
Common hepatic duct
Cystic duct
Stomach
Common bile duct
Bile
Duodenal ampulla

Bile ducts

Visceral surface

Fibrous appendix of the liver
Ligamentum venosum — Inferior vena cava — Ligament of the inferior vena cava
Caudate lobe
Left lobe
Right lobe
Portal vein
Hepatic artery
Bile duct
Round ligament of the liver
Quadrate lobe
Gallbladder

Liver lobule function

To the inferior vena cava
Central vein
Hepatic artery
Liver lobule
Branch of bile duct
Branch of portal vein

■ Bile collects in the common bile duct
■ Blood from the digestive system
■ Oxygenated blood from the heart
■ Deoxygenated and processed blood returning to the heart

The liver possesses the unique capability to regenerate to within 5 to 10% of its original weight after damage from viral or toxic injuries or partial surgical removal. Hepatocytes, stimulated by growth factors after injury, replicate under a process of controlled cell division to restore the liver's volume.

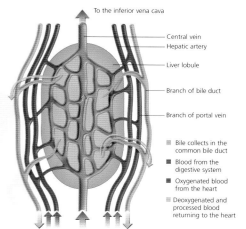

Vessel
Sinusoid
Red blood cell
White blood cell
Kupffer cell
Portal triad
Hepatic artery
Bile canaliculi
Fat storing cell
Branch of portal vein
Hepatocyte
Branch of bile duct
Bile canaliculi (cross-section)

Enlarged view of the liver lobule

■ **Venous blood** *(filtered)*
■ **Portal blood** *(unfiltered)*

Central vein
Sinusoids
Interlobular septum
Central vein
Liver lobule

Portal triad
■ Hepatic artery
■ Branch of portal vein
■ Branch of bile duct

Structure of the liver

The two lobes of the liver are divided into thousands of functional microscopic units called **lobules**. Blood is delivered to the lobules via the liver's two sources of blood supply: the **hepatic artery**, which carries oxygen-rich blood from the heart, and the **hepatic portal vein**, carrying nutrients from the digestive system.

Each lobule contains layers of **hepatocytes** (liver cells) arranged in cords or sheets radiating out from a central vein. The **hepatic sinusoids** form tunnels or spaces between groups of these layers. Lobules are polygonal in shape, with six **portal triads** at the corners that each contain three vessels: a branch of the hepatic vein, a branch of the hepatic artery and a bile duct. Blood flows into the sinusoids from the portal triads, eventually reaching the **central veins**. Bile flows out of the lobule toward the portal triads through the **bile canaliculi**.

Injury to the liver can result in restricted blood flow through the hepatic portal system, causing portal hypertension, a condition commonly associated with cirrhosis.

PLATE 20

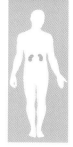

The Urinary System

The urinary system is responsible for three major functions in the body: **removing wastes, maintaining normal water volume,** and **controlling acid-base balance** in the bloodstream. The individual components of the urinary system (bladder, kidneys, ureters and urethra) each play an important role in these processes.

Urine formation begins within tiny functional units of the kidneys called **nephrons**. A complex, three-step process of **filtration, reabsorption** and **secretion** removes metabolic wastes, allows important substances such as glucose and water to be passed back into the blood, and eliminates toxins such as drugs and ammonia. The filtrate that results from this process is eventually diluted with water to produce urine.

Urine from the kidneys is pushed towards the bladder through narrow tubes called **ureters**. The bladder stores the urine until stretching of the muscle walls triggers the impulse to urinate, typically when the bladder contains about 200 mL of urine. Two sphincters regulate the release of urine through the urethra, a thin tube that leads from the bladder to the outside of the body.

Structure of the kidneys

The kidneys are located on each side of the spine at the back of the abdominal cavity. Each kidney is approximately 4 to 5 inches long and connects to the bladder via a narrow muscular tube called a **ureter**. We are normally born with a pair of kidneys; however, we can survive with a single kidney.

Each kidney is supported by a layer of connective tissue (**renal fascia**) and surrounded by a **fatty renal capsule**. Within the kidney are two main regions. The outer rim is the **renal cortex**, which contains the **nephrons**, tiny microscopic units that filter blood (*see below*). The inner region is the **renal medulla**. It consists of many cone-shaped structures (**renal pyramids**) that transport urine to the calyces, cup-shaped cavities in the center of the kidney. The calyces drain into the **renal sinus**, a central chamber that connects directly to the ureter.

Functions of the kidneys

The primary function of the kidneys is to filter and eliminate excess water and waste products from the blood. In addition, the kidneys help maintain normal blood pressure by excreting excess sodium and secreting the enzyme **renin**. The kidneys also secrete **erythropoietin**, a hormone essential for the production of red blood cells, and produce active **vitamin D (calcitriol)** to help maintain healthy bones.

The nephron

Each kidney contains more than a million nephrons, the microscopic units located in the outer renal cortex. Nephrons regulate levels of water and soluble substances in the body by filtering the blood; reabsorbing water, glucose and valuable ions such as potassium and sodium; and excreting excess water and waste products.

A single nephron is made up of four components: the **renal corpuscle**, the **proximal convoluted tubule**, the **loop of Henle** and the **distal convoluted tubule**. Blood is first filtered in the renal corpuscle before passing to the proximal tubule, where water and other usable substances are reabsorbed and returned to the bloodstream. The filtrate enters the loop of Henle, and sodium, potassium and chloride are pumped out. In the final stages, additional sodium is removed within the distal tubule and exchanged for potassium and acid. Concentrated urine leaves the nephron via a **collecting duct**.

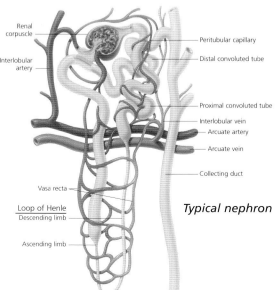

Typical nephron

Renal corpuscle
Interlobular artery
Peritubular capillary
Distal convoluted tube
Proximal convoluted tube
Interlobular vein
Arcuate artery
Arcuate vein
Collecting duct
Vasa recta
Loop of Henle
Descending limb
Ascending limb

Renal corpuscle

The renal corpuscle consists of two parts:

- **Glomerular capsule**, a hollow, cup-shaped bulb that connects to the renal tubule
- The **glomerulus**, a rounded cluster of capillaries where blood cells and larger molecules are filtered

As blood enters the glomerulus at a high pressure, blood is filtered through tiny pores in the glomerular capillaries. The remaining clear fluid containing ions, amino acids, glucose and other substances enters the **glomerular capsule**, which passes the fluid to the upper part of the renal tubule (PCT) to begin tubular reabsorption.

Adjacent to the renal corpuscle and distal convoluted tubule are specialized cells called the **juxtaglomerular apparatus**. These cells monitor blood pressure as it enters the kidney and react to reduced blood flow by secreting renin, an enzyme stored in the kidney. Renin increases blood pressure by constricting blood vessels and triggering increased reabsorption of sodium and chloride to raise fluid volumes.

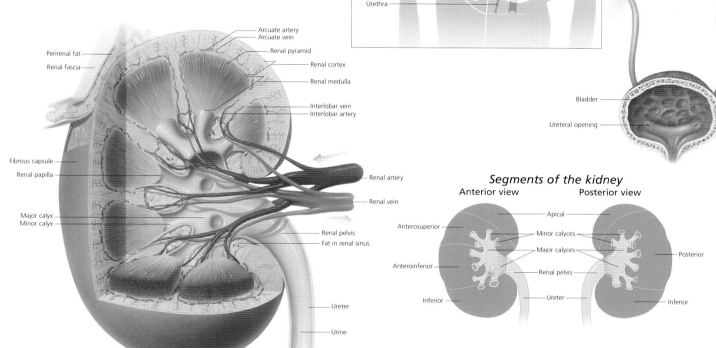

Kidney
Renal artery
Renal vein
Ureter

Female pelvis

Ovary
Uterus
Bladder
Urethra

Male pelvis

Bladder
Prostate
Urethra

Bladder
Ureteral opening

Arcuate artery
Arcuate vein
Renal pyramid
Renal cortex
Renal medulla
Interlobar vein
Interlobar artery
Perirenal fat
Renal fascia
Fibrous capsule
Renal papilla
Renal artery
Renal vein
Major calyx
Minor calyx
Renal pelvis
Fat in renal sinus
Ureter
Urine

Segments of the kidney

Anterior view   Posterior view

Anterosuperior
Anteroinferior
Inferior
Apical
Minor calyces
Major calyces
Renal pelvis
Ureter
Posterior
Inferior

Filtrate formation

Glomerular capsule
Efferent arteriole
Afferent arteriole
Collecting tube
Water and other substances
Urine
Distal convoluted tube
Filtrate flow
Water and other substances
Blood flow

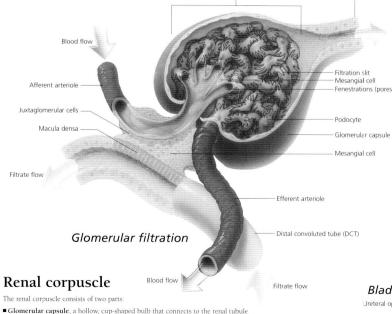

Glomerular filtration

Glomerulus
Proximal convoluted tube (PCT)
Blood flow
Afferent arteriole
Juxtaglomerular cells
Macula densa
Filtrate flow
Filtration slit
Mesangial cell
Fenestrations (pores)
Podocyte
Glomerular capsule
Mesangial cell
Efferent arteriole
Distal convoluted tube (DCT)
Blood flow
Filtrate flow

How urine is produced

The kidneys process an average of 200 quarts of blood daily, eventually excreting only about 2 quarts of extra water and waste products as urine. Urine production begins when blood enters the nephrons. After a complex process of reabsorption and secretion along the renal tubule, concentrated urine containing water and wastes such as sodium and urea (a by-product of toxic ammonia products formed in the liver) leaves the collecting ducts. The urine then drains into the calyces of the kidney and enters the ureters, which push small amounts of urine in low-pressure waves to the bladder.

Key stages of urine formation

- **Filtration** — filtering of water, waste products, sodium, glucose and other chemicals
- **Reabsorption** — movement of usable substances back to the bloodstream
- **Secretion** — transport of waste materials from capillaries around the renal tubule back into the distal tubule for removal with the urine

Bladder

Ureteral opening
Detrusor muscle
Neck of urinary bladder
Internal urethral sphincter

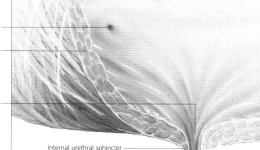

PLATE 21

The Lymphatic System

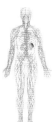

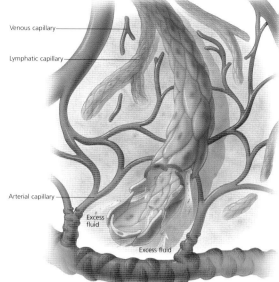

Venous capillary
Lymphatic capillary
Arterial capillary
Excess fluid
Excess fluid

What is the lymphatic system?

The **lymphatic system** is an extensive network of vessels and nodes that forms a central part of the body's defenses against illness and injury. Foreign materials such as bacteria or dead cells are collected and transported through the **lymph vessels**, where they are filtered by the **lymph nodes**. The lymph vessels also drain excess fluid from the body's tissues, forming a fluid called **lymph**, and carry substances such as cholesterol and fat-soluble vitamins from the gastrointestinal system to the bloodstream.

The lymphatic system contains millions of **lymphocytes**, cells that trigger immune responses, target and destroy pathogens, and produce **antibodies**, proteins that inactivate specific antigens. The lymphatic system is closely integrated with two kinds of lymphatic organs and tissues throughout the body.

Primary lymphatic organs. The **bone marrow** produces cells that divide and mature to become B lymphocytes, or migrate to the **thymus** to develop into T lymphocytes. Each type of lymphocyte plays a specific role in immune response.

Secondary lymphatic organs. Most immune responses actually take place in the secondary lymphatic organs and tissues such as the **lymph nodes**, **spleen**, **tonsils** and **mucosa-associated lymphatic tissue (MALT)**, located throughout the linings of the gastrointestinal, urinary, reproductive and respiratory systems.

Right lymphatic drainage
Left lymphatic drainage

Right lymphatic duct — Left lymphatic duct
— Thymus
Axillary nodes — Thoracic duct
Cisterna chyli
— Spleen
Lumbar nodes
Inguinal nodes
Popliteal nodes
Lymphatics

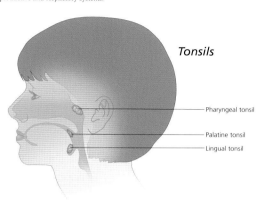

Tonsils

Pharyngeal tonsil
Palatine tonsil
Lingual tonsil

Lymph and lymph vessels

Lymph vessels begin as microscopic capillaries in intercellular spaces throughout the body and converge to form larger lymphatic vessels similar to veins. The lymph capillaries absorb excess fluid filtered from the blood to provide the tissues with oxygen and nutrients. Once inside the lymph vessels, this clear, watery **interstitial fluid** becomes known as **lymph**. While most interstitial fluid is reabsorbed by the blood vessels, approximately 15% returns to the blood system through the lymph vessels. This function helps to maintain the fluid volume of the body.

All lymph passing through the lymphatic system is filtered by the lymph nodes lining the vessels. The lymph eventually flows into large channels called the **thoracic** and **right lymphatic ducts** and drains back into the bloodstream through the **subclavian veins**.

Lymphoid intestinal tissue

Groups of lymphatic nodules known as **mucosa-associated lymphatic tissue (MALT)** are located throughout the mucosal linings of many areas of the body. In the gastrointestinal tract, concentrations of lymphatic nodules are referred to as **gut-associated lymphoid tissue (GALT)**. This important secondary lymphatic tissue includes large specialized aggregates called **Peyer's patches**, and is believed to play an important role in defending the gut from harmful bacteria and other foreign substances.

Lymph node

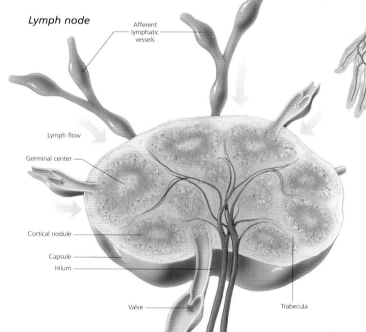

Afferent lymphatic vessels
Lymph flow
Germinal center
Cortical nodule
Capsule
Hilum
Valve
Trabecula
Efferent lymphatic vessel
Vein
Artery
Lymph flow

Lymph nodes

The lymphatic vessels are lined with hundreds of tiny bean-shaped organs called **lymph nodes**. Although they are scattered throughout the body, large clusters of lymph nodes are concentrated near specific areas such as the **mammary glands** and **groin**. Lymph nodes act as a barrier to infection by scavenging bacteria and other foreign materials from the lymph collected from the organs and tissues before it is returned to the bloodstream.

Each lymph node is surrounded by a thick capsule of fibrous tissue and densely packed with lymphocytes, including T cells, antibody-secreting B cells, and scavenging cells called **macrophages**, which ingest foreign matter and debris trapped by specialized fibers within the node's lymphatic sinuses.

Swollen lymph nodes often indicate the presence of infection or cancer.

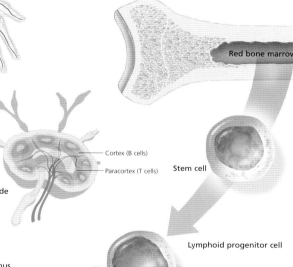

Red bone marrow
Cortex (B cells)
Paracortex (T cells)
Stem cell
Lymph node
Lymphoid progenitor cell
Thymus
NK cell
B cell
T cell

Inflammatory and immune responses

There are two basic kinds of immunity. **Innate** or **nonspecific immunity** is present at birth and involves white blood cells including **monocytes**, **neutrophils** and **eosinophils**, and certain lymphocytes called **NK (natural killer) cells**. These cells play similar roles in attacking and destroying bacteria and other foreign substances. Inflammation is a nonspecific response to invasion by pathogens, injury such as abrasions or cell disturbances, and severe temperature.

Through **specific** or **adaptive immunity**, the body learns and remembers the responses needed to destroy specific antigens. Lymphocytes play a key role in specific immune responses because they are long-lived cells that "remember" the specific antigens they encounter and can react quickly and directly each time the antigen enters the body. Specific immunity involves two different types of responses:

■ **Cell-mediated responses.** This process triggers killer, or cytotoxic, T lymphocytes to directly attack the antigen and is typically targeted pathogens that invade host cells, such as viruses and some cancer cells.

■ **Antibody-mediated responses.** Antibodies synthesized from **B cells** are produced to inactivate the attacking antigen. This response works primarily against pathogens such as bacteria that multiply in body fluids without entering the cells.

Complement proteins. The antimicrobial activity of complement proteins enhances or complements the body's immune, allergic and inflammatory reactions. Complement proteins are found in the blood plasma and on the plasma membranes.

Immune system disorders

Immune disorders occur when the immune system mistakenly reacts against itself and destroys healthy cells and tissues (autoimmune disorders and allergic reactions), or fails to generate sufficient immune response to protect the body from invading pathogens (immunodeficiency).

Autoimmune disorders can occur as a result of injuries, viruses, radiation, or by ingesting certain drugs or other foreign substances. They can also result from a malfunction of the B lymphocytes, which produce abnormal antibodies. Autoimmune disorders include **Type 1 diabetes**, **lupus**, **pernicious anemia** and **Graves' disease**.

Allergic reactions involve an excessive immune reaction to a normally harmless substance. Allergic reactions can be caused by exposure to allergens ranging from **pollen** and **dust** to **drugs**, **food** and **animal dander**. Most allergic symptoms are mild, but some can trigger asthma or sudden anaphylactic reactions requiring immediate treatment.

Immunodeficiency disorders impair the body's ability to defend itself against pathogens, resulting in abnormally frequent or severe infections. Immunodeficiency disorders may be congenital or develop as a result of a secondary disease or infection, such as **human immunodeficiency virus (HIV)**. Immunodeficiency can also be caused by **malnutrition** and **immunosuppressant drugs**.

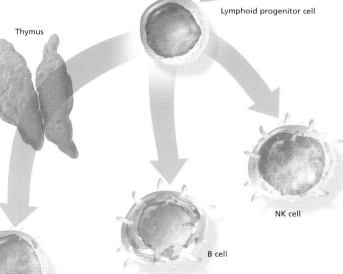

Formation of lymphocytes

All lymphocytes originate as **stem cells** during fetal development. Specific lymphocyte growth and production takes place in the primary lymphatic organs (bone marrow and thymus gland), where the stem cells divide and mature into B and T cells.

B lymphocytes remain in the bone marrow and develop unique receptors targeted to specific antigens. B cells secrete antibodies, large protein molecules that combine with and destroy invading antigens. B cells ultimately form millions of different kinds of antibodies, each with specific antigen-targeting properties.

T lymphocytes begin in the bone marrow and migrate to the thymus gland, located between the lungs and behind the breastbone. They divide rapidly, eventually developing reactive properties against millions of different antigens. Through a complex process within the thymus, T cells become "self-recognizing" so they react only against outside antigens, not against other lymphocytes. Killer, or cytotoxic, T lymphocytes recognize and destroy infected or abnormal cells.

NK (natural killer) cells are lymphocytes related to T cells. NK cells require no previous activation, providing a nonspecific response to virus-infected and malignant cells.

PLATE 22

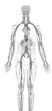

The Endocrine System

What is the endocrine system?

The endocrine system is made up of organs and glands that produce **hormones**, internal chemical messengers that regulate and control functions within the body. Hormones are secreted into the bloodstream and trigger activity within a specific organ or tissue by binding to designated receptors to transmit information.

The endocrine system regulates body processes including metabolism and energy balance, reproduction, growth and development, smooth and cardiac muscle contraction, and blood volumes of substances such as sodium and glucose. The activities of the endocrine system are closely coordinated with the nervous system.

The major organs and glands of the endocrine system include the **hypothalamus, thymus, pancreas, ovaries**, and **testes**, as well as the **pituitary, pineal, thyroid, adrenal,** and **parathyroid glands**.

Thymus

The **thymus** produces the thymic hormones, which promote the development of white blood cells called T lymphocytes. The thymus is located between the lungs and behind the breastbone. It is very large at birth but shrinks as thymic tissue is replaced by fat and connective tissue after puberty.

Adult
Juvenile

Heart

Many different endocrine hormones are essential to the function of the cardiovascular system. **Epinephrine** and **norepinephrine** increase heart rate and muscle contractions. **Erythropoietin (EPO)** promotes red blood cell production. **Aldosterone** and **antidiuretic** hormones **(ADH)** increase the volume of blood.

The endocrine system and hormones

The release of hormones is controlled by **feedback** from different parts of the body. Bursts of hormones are released into the blood in response to signals from the nervous system, as well as by changes in blood chemistry and the actions of other hormones. When sufficient levels of a specific hormone reach the target tissue, stimulation of the hormone-producing organ stops and hormone blood levels decrease.

1. Initial stimulus from hypothalamus

4. Feedback to the pituitary

3. Hormonal response

2. From pituitary through vascular system to target organ

Target organ

Action of hormones

There are many hormones in the circulatory system at the same time. Specific hormones attach to cells having a certain receptor. These cells are called "target" cells. If a cell does not have a receptor, the hormone doesn't connect, and the cells don't respond.

Hormone receptor
Hormones
Blood vessel
Hormone
Target cell

P neal gland
Hypothalamus
P tuitary gland

The pineal gland

The **pineal gland** (attached to the third ventricle of the brain) produces **melatonin**, which regulates the body's biological clock and helps to control sleep patterns.

Thyroid
Parathyroid (Posterior)

Thyroid and parathyroids

The **thyroid** gland is found posterior to the larynx. Thyroid hormones influence rate of metabolism as well as body temperature, protein synthesis and cholesterol secretion. The four **parathyroid** glands attached to the thyroid produce parathyroid hormone (PTH), which regulates blood levels of electrolytes (i.e., calcium, magnesium and phosphate).

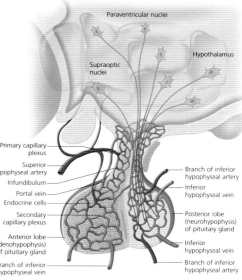

Paraventricular nuclei
Supraoptic nuclei
Hypothalamus
Primary capillary plexus
Superior hypophyseal artery
Infundibulum
Portal vein
Endocrine cells
Secondary capillary plexus
Anterior lobe (adenohypophysis) of pituitary gland
Branch of inferior hypophyseal vein
Branch of inferior hypophyseal artery
Inferior hypophyseal vein
Posterior lobe (neurohypophysis) of pituitary gland
Inferior hypophyseal vein
Branch of inferior hypophyseal artery

The hypothalamus and pituitary gland

The **hypothalamus** is a small region of the brain that coordinates the nervous and endocrine systems. The hypothalamus secretes a variety of major hormones and also dictates the function of the pituitary gland. In turn, the pituitary produces the hormones that control the functions of most of the body's other endocrine glands.

The **pituitary gland** itself is a tiny structure located within the base of the brain. It has two distinct regions. The anterior pituitary synthesizes six major hormones, including **human growth hormone (HGH)** and **thyroid stimulating hormone (TSH)**. The posterior pituitary secretes **oxytocin**, important in labor and breast feeding, and **antidiuretic hormone (ADH)**, which controls water secretion by the kidneys.

Digestive system

The complex process of digestion is regulated by hormones produced in the gut, including **gastrin, cholecystokinin, secretin,** and **gastric inhibitory peptide (GIP)**.

Adrenal gland

The two adrenal glands, located just above the kidneys, produce hormones that regulate salt and water balance **(aldosterone)**; support the immune system and influence mood **(dehydroepiandrosterone or DHEA)**; combat stress and maintain blood sugar and blood pressure **(cortisol)**; and stimulate the nervous system and increase heart rate **(epinephrine** and **norepinephrine)**.

Kidney

Renin and **angiotensin** are secreted by the kidneys to produce **angiotensin II**, a hormone that raises blood pressure by causing constriction of the blood vessels and also stimulates the secretion of the hormone **aldosterone** (a process called the **renin-angiotensin-aldosterone pathway)**. Red blood cell production is stimulated by the release of **erythropoietin (EPO)**.

Pancreas

The **pancreatic islets** (Islets of Langerhans) within the pancreas are responsible for secreting **glucagon**, which raises blood sugar levels. They also produce **insulin**, which lowers blood sugar levels and controls the metabolism of sugar, protein, and fat.

Insulin
Blood glucose level
Glucagon
Epinephrine cortisol
Human growth hormone

Function of insulin

During digestion, sugar is absorbed into the bloodstream and stimulates the production of insulin in the pancreas. Insulin allows glucose to diffuse from the blood into essential body tissues, particularly the skeletal muscles. Insulin also controls blood sugar by promoting protein synthesis in the cells and regulating glucose and glycogen conversion in the liver.

Reproductive organs

Testes

Testosterone, the primary male sex hormone, is produced in the male reproductive glands or testes. Testosterone stimulates the growth and development of the male sex organs and secondary sex characteristics (e.g. it also controls the production of sperm). Additional hormones secreted by the pituitary, **luteinizing hormone (LH)** and **follicle stimulating hormone (FSH)**, are important for the production of testosterone and sperm cells.

Ovaries

The ovaries produce the female sex hormones. **Estrogens** are responsible for the development of the female reproductive structures, sexual characteristics, and breast development. **Progesterone** prepares the uterine lining for implantation of a fertilized egg and is necessary for breast milk production.

The ovaries also produce **relaxin** and **inhibin**, hormones that direct uterine muscle relaxation and regulate the menstrual cycle.

Menstrual cycle

The menstrual cycle is controlled by gonadotropin-releasing hormone (GnRH), secreted by the hypothalamus. During the first two weeks, GnRH directs the release of follicle stimulating hormone (FSH) from the anterior pituitary, stimulating the growth of follicles in the ovaries and the secretion of estrogen. Around 14 days, luteinizing hormone (LH) released by the anterior pituitary stimulates the release of a ripened egg (ovum) and production of estrogens, progesterone, relaxin and inhibin by the corpus luteum (endocrine tissue formed in the follicle after the release of the ovum).

If fertilization does not occur, declining estrogen and progesterone levels decrease blood supply to the lining of the uterus. The lining sloughs off during menstruation, resulting in the menstrual flow.

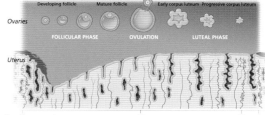

Developing follicle
Mature follicle
Early corpus luteum
Progressive corpus luteum
Ovaries
FOLLICULAR PHASE
OVULATION
LUTEAL PHASE
Uterus
Days 0   4   14   26

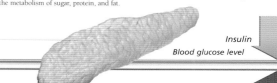

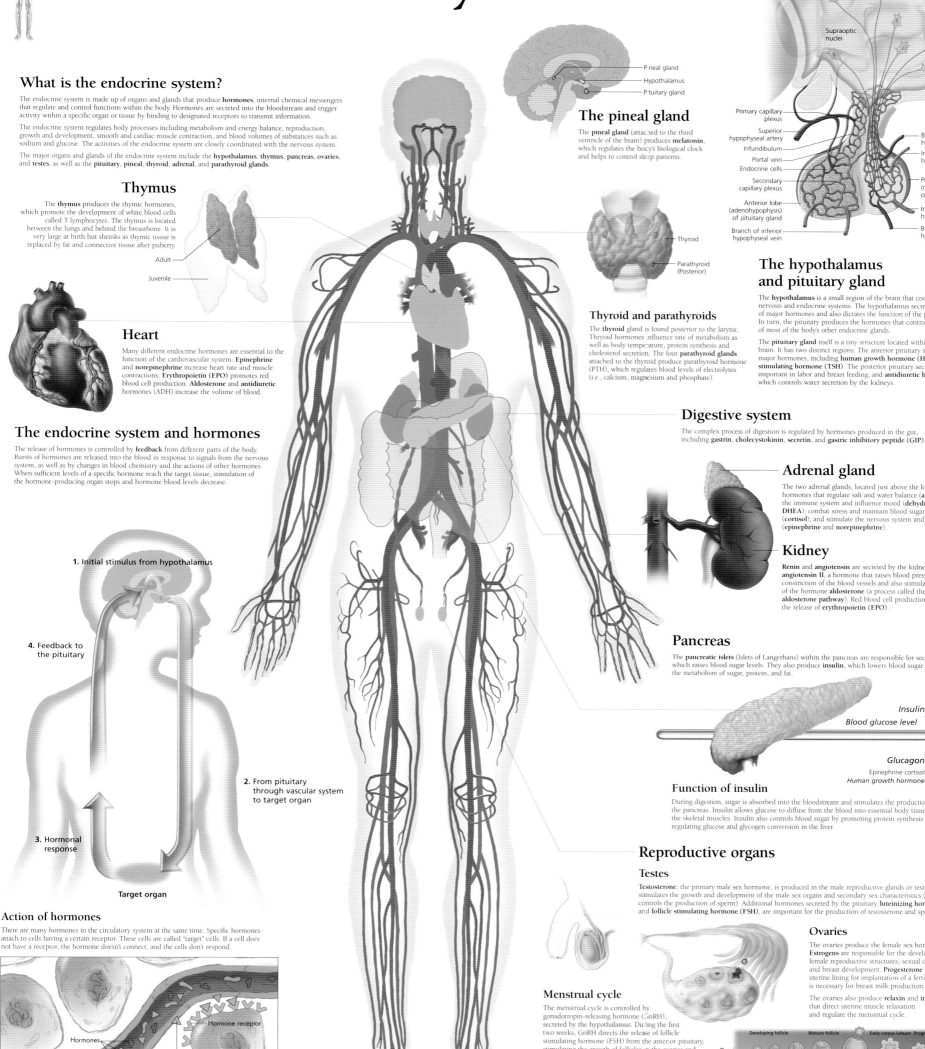

PLATE 23

The Male Reproductive System

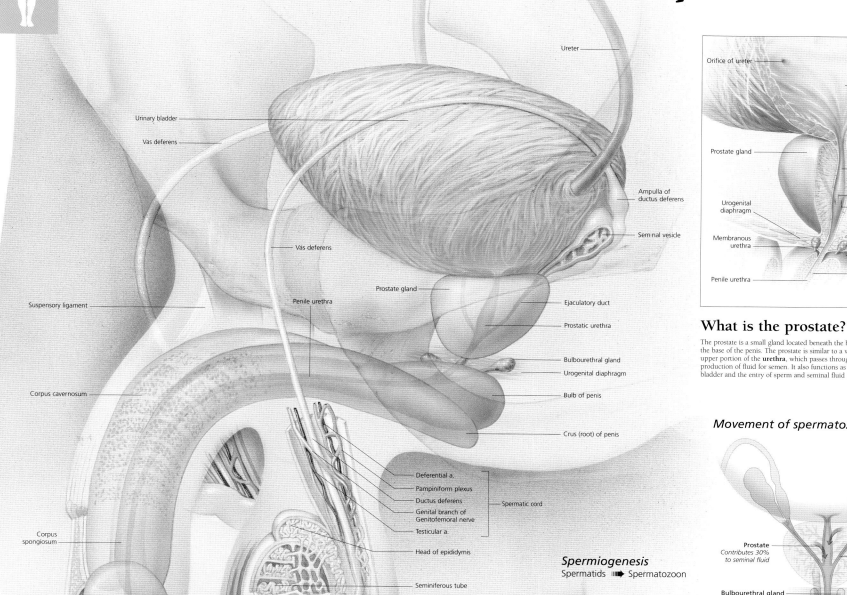

Ureter

Urinary bladder

Vas deferens

Ampulla of ductus deferens

Vas deferens

Seminal vesicle

Suspensory ligament

Prostate gland

Ejaculatory duct

Penile urethra

Prostatic urethra

Corpus cavernosum

Bulbourethral gland

Urogenital diaphragm

Bulb of penis

Crus (root) of penis

Corpus spongiosum

Deferential a.
Pampiniform plexus
Ductus deferens
Genital branch of Genitofemoral nerve
Testicular a.

Spermatic cord

Head of epididymis

Navicular fossa

Seminiferous tube

Prepuce

Body of epididymis

External urethral opening

Glans

Skin
Dartos muscle
Superficial scrotal fascia
Cremaster muscle

Tail of epididymis

Testis (covered by visceral layer of tunica vaginalis)

The Prostate
Anterior view (sectioned)

Orifice of ureter

Urinary bladder

Prostate gland

Seminal vesicle

Ejaculatory duct (shaded)

Prostatic urethra

Urogenital diaphragm

Prostatic utricle

Membranous urethra

Orifice of ejaculatory duct

Penile urethra

Bulbourethral gland

Bulb of penis

Opening of bulbourethral duct

What is the prostate?

The prostate is a small gland located beneath the bladder and just in front of the rectum, behind the base of the penis. The prostate is similar to a walnut in both shape and size and surrounds the upper portion of the **urethra**, which passes through it. The primary purpose of the prostate is the production of fluid for semen. It also functions as a valve, preventing the leakage of urine from the bladder and the entry of sperm and seminal fluid into the bladder.

Movement of spermatozoa

Seminal vesicle *Contributes 60% to seminal fluid*

Prostate *Contributes 30% to seminal fluid*

Ejaculatory duct

Ductus deferens

Bulbourethral gland *Contributes 5% to seminal fluid*

Penile urethra

Spermatozoa movement by peristaltic action of the ductus deferens

Ejaculate

Head of epididymis

Epididymis and sustentacular cells Contribute 5% to seminal fluid

Tail of epididymis

Accessory glands
- Seminal vesicles
- Prostate
- Bulbourethral glands

Spermiogenesis
Spermatids ⟹ Spermatozoon

Nucleus

Mitochondria

Acrosomal vesicle

Spermatid

Acrosomal vesicle

Flagellum

Male reproductive system

The adult male reproductive system is comprised of two primary external structures, the **testes** and the **penis**. The testes are a pair of organs approximately 1.5 inches in length and 1 inch in diameter. They are each divided into hundreds of tiny compartments or **lobules** containing the **seminiferous tubules**, tightly coiled structures where **spermatogenesis** and **spermiogenesis** take place.

The testes are encased in a protective sachlike structure called the **scrotum**, which provides support and regulates the position of the testes relative to the body. The scrotum is divided into two compartments that separate the testes from each other, preventing injury or infection on one side from affecting the other. The inner muscle layers of the scrotum react to changes in external temperature to maintain the proper temperature within the testes for spermatogenesis. The testes are relaxed and lowered during warm temperatures and contracted and elevated when cold.

Testosterone is produced within the testes by specialized cells known as **interstitial cells**. Testosterone is the male hormone responsible for maintaining the structure and function of the sex organs and promoting the development of male secondary sex characteristics.

Vascularization

Cremasteric a., v.

Deferential a., v.

Inferior vesical a., v.

Subcutaneous median dorsal a., v.

Perineal a., v.

Deep dorsal vein of penis

Testicular a.

Deferential a., v.
Pampiniform plexus

Dorsal arteries of penis

Anterior scrotal a., v.

Posterior scrotal a., v.

Vasectomy

Urinary bladder

Vas deferens

Cut and suture

Cut and suture

Epididymis

Testis

Vasectomy is a surgical procedure that involves cutting and sealing the vas deferens, or ducts that transport sperm from the testes. Small incisions are made in the skin of the scrotum and approximately one half-inch is removed from the vas deferens in each testis. The ends are sutured or cauterized and placed back in the scrotum. It is possible to reverse the procedure by reattaching the vas deferens, but more extensive surgery is required and only 30 to 40 percent of men who undergo vasectomy reversal may be able to successfully father children.

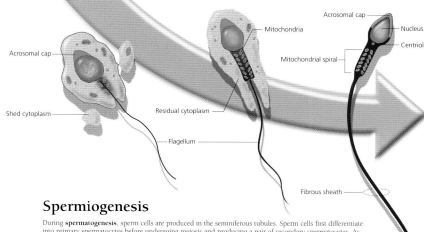

Acrosomal cap

Mitochondria

Acrosomal cap

Nucleus

Mitochondrial spiral

Centriole

Shed cytoplasm

Residual cytoplasm

Flagellum

Fibrous sheath

Spermatozoon

Spermiogenesis

During **spermatogenesis**, sperm cells are produced in the seminiferous tubules. Sperm cells first differentiate into primary spermatocytes before undergoing meiosis and producing a pair of secondary spermatocytes. As each secondary spermatocyte divides, a pair of spermatids is produced. In the next phase, **spermiogenesis**, the spermatids are embedded within large cells called **sustentacular cells**, where they continue to mature. Spermatids undergo a dramatic change in form during spermiogenesis, gradually developing the structure and appearance of functional **spermatozoa**. Newly produced spermatozoa detach from the sustentacular cells and are transported to the **epididymis**, a coiled thin-walled tube within the scrotum that connects the testis to the **vas deferens** (the duct through which sperm travel to the prostate before ejaculation).

PLATE 24

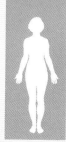

The Female Reproductive System

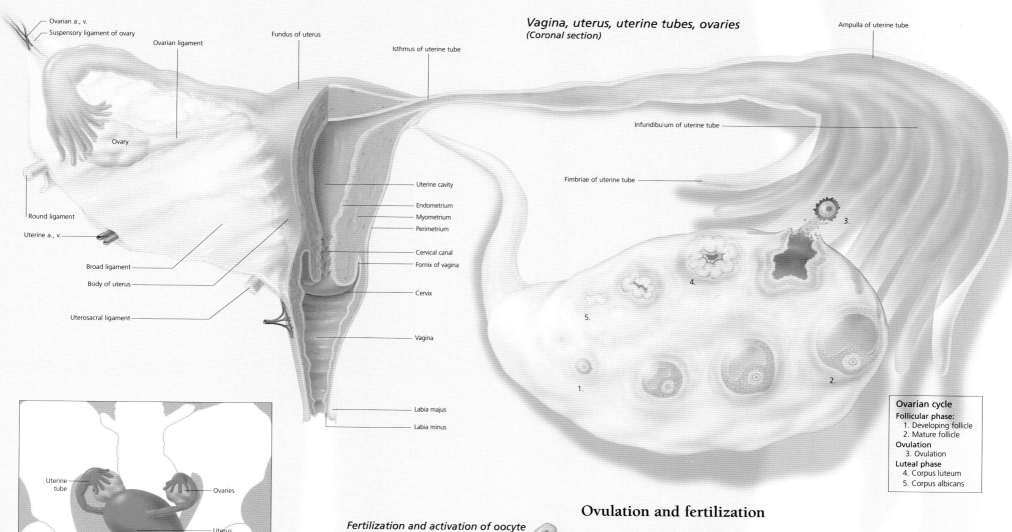

Vagina, uterus, uterine tubes, ovaries
(Coronal section)

Ovarian a., v.
Suspensory ligament of ovary
Ovarian ligament
Fundus of uterus
Isthmus of uterine tube
Ampulla of uterine tube

Ovary

Infundibulum of uterine tube

Fimbriae of uterine tube

Round ligament
Uterine a., v.

Uterine cavity
Endometrium
Myometrium
Perimetrium

Broad ligament
Body of uterus

Cervical canal
Fornix of vagina

Uterosacral ligament

Cervix

Vagina

1.
2.
3.
4.
5.

Labia majus
Labia minus

Ovarian cycle
Follicular phase:
1. Developing follicle
2. Mature follicle
Ovulation
3. Ovulation
Luteal phase
4. Corpus luteum
5. Corpus albicans

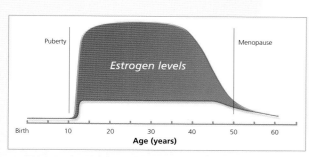

Uterine tube
Ovaries
Uterus
Bladder
Vagina

Female reproductive system

The internal structures of the adult female reproductive system include the vagina, cervix, uterus, ovaries and uterine tubes. These structures form a pathway allowing the release of **ova** (egg cells), fertilization by **sperm** and delivery of a developed fetus.

The **vagina** is a muscular tube approximately 3 to 4 inches long. It extends from the external genital organs to the **cervix**, the lower part of the uterus. A channel through the cervix allows the passage of sperm and menstrual discharge.

The **uterus**, a hollow pear-shaped organ with muscular walls that contract during childbirth, consists of three sections: the cervix, a tapered middle section known as the **corpus** (main body) and the wide **fundus** at the top of the uterus. The inner lining of the corpus is the **endometrium**, which thickens during each menstrual cycle in preparation for implantation by a fertilized egg. This lining is shed during menstruation if fertilization does not occur.

The **ovaries** are located on each side of the uterus. These small oval glands are similar to an almond in size and shape. They are responsible for producing ova as well as the female sex hormones **estrogen** and **progesterone**. The ovaries are connected to the uterus by the fallopian tubes, narrow ducts approximately 2 to 3 inches in length that provide a passageway for the ova to reach the uterus. Fertilization normally occurs in the uterine tubes.

Ovulation and fertilization

Fertilization and activation of oocyte

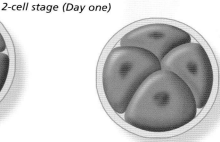

2-cell stage (Day one)

4-cell stage (Day two)

Ovulation is the release of a single mature ovum from one of the ovaries, which is triggered by a sudden rise in the blood level of the gonadotrophic hormone LH. The ovum travels down the uterine tube and enters the uterine cavity. An unfertilized ovum passes out of the body through the vagina. Ovulation normally occurs around day 14 of the cycle.

Fertilization is the fusion of genetic material from a mature ovum with that from a mature sperm to produce a fertilized egg (or zygote). Fertilization normally occurs in the uterine tube. The zygote begins to divide as it travels down the uterine tube towards the uterus, eventually forming an embryo that may successfully implant into the endometrium.

Nucleus
Polar body
Zona pellucida
Corona radiata

Oocyte at ovulation

What is estrogen?

Estrogen is the female sex hormone. There are actually several different estrogens, the most important being **estradiol**. Estrogens are produced in the **ovaries**, which are located in the lateral walls of the pelvis on either side of the **uterus** (womb). The two ovaries produce female sex cells (the ova or 'eggs') and hormones (estrogens). The ovaries do not begin to produce estrogens until the onset of puberty. Estrogens are responsible for the appearance of female **secondary sexual characteristics**, which enable a young woman to achieve full reproductive fertility (e.g. growth of the reproductive organs, onset of menstrual periods, etc.).

Estrogens affect the female reproductive organs and other parts of the body –
- **Genital tract:** estrogens stimulate a favorable environment for the survival of sperm during the **menstrual cycle**
- **Breast tissue:** estrogens stimulate the growth of non-glandular breast tissue
- **Heart:** estrogens improve circulation and prevent high blood pressure
- **Skeleton:** estrogens help retain calcium in the bones

Puberty
Menopause
Estrogen levels
Birth 10 20 30 40 50 60
Age (years)

What is the menstrual cycle?

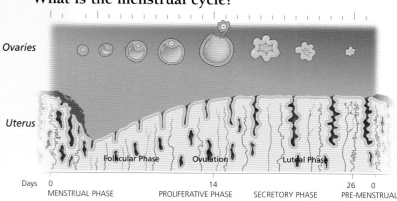

Ovaries
Uterus

Days 0 14 26 0
MENSTRUAL PHASE PROLIFERATIVE PHASE SECRETORY PHASE PRE-MENSTRUAL
Follicular Phase Ovulation Luteal Phase

The **menstrual cycle** refers to the sequence of events that occurs in the cell layers lining the uterus (womb), called the **endometrial layer** or **endometrium**; it normally lasts for approximately 28 days. The purpose of the menstrual cycle is to prepare the uterus for possible pregnancy. It is intimately linked to events occurring in the ovary that prepare a mature ovum (or egg cell) for release (ovulation) and possible fertilization; this is known as the ovarian cycle. Hormones produced in the ovaries, namely **estrogens** and **progesterone**, control the menstrual cycle. Hormones produced in the brain control the ovarian cycle; these hormones are called **gonadotrophins** (LH and FSH).

During menstruation the cells lining the uterus (endometrium) become detached from the uterine wall and fall off. This is accompanied by bleeding and normally lasts around 5 days. The tissue pieces and blood pass into the vagina and out of the body. Menstruation marks the **beginning** of the menstrual cycle.

PLATE 25